For centuries, millions throughout the world have used the systems and disciplines of Yoga to attain physical and mental youthfulness, find improved health, and discover a new and thrilling awareness of themselves and the Universal consciousness.

Rejuvenation Through Yoga brings together the basic teachings of Hatha Yoga. It presents specially developed exercises for use when swimming and diving, in a completely illustrated, simple-to-use form.

Rejuvenation Through Yoga can be your guide to a new and more rewarding life. It can bring improved health and the joy of youthful vigor to anyone who will devote a few minutes a day to this age-old system of health and hygiene.

Also by Goldie Lipson

BEYOND YOGA

REJUVENATION THROUGH YOGA

Goldie Lipson
A.E. - N.A.W.A.

Based on the Teachings of
RAMMURTI S. MISHRA, M.D.
East-West Guru

Illustrated by the Author

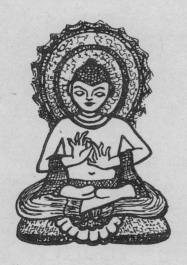

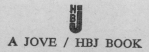

A JOVE / HBJ BOOK

Five previous printings
First Jove/HBJ edition published March 1978

Printed in the United States of America

Jove/HBJ books are published by Jove Publications, Inc.
(Harcourt Brace Jovanovich),
757 Third Avenue, New York, N.Y. 10017

Contents

RAMMURTI S. MISHRA, M.A., M.D.

Dr. Rammurti S. Mishra dedicates his life and energy to the service of the world through the teaching of Universal Principle and Law. A qualified Sanskrit scholar, Dr. Mishra has lectured extensively in many countries and has had his works published. He has done a great deal of research in the field of medicine; his efforts span his career which began as chief of his service at the Podar Hospital, Bombay, India and includes his service on the staff at the Hospital for Incurable Diseases at New York University Hospital where he specialized in endocrinology. He commenced his study of Psychiatry at Rhode Island State Hospital, near Providence. After the completion of one year, he transferred to McGill University, Montreal, Canada for more extensive training in the field of psychiatry. Following this, Dr. Mishra joined the staff at Bellevue Hospital, New York City as a neurosurgeon. He has been connected with New York University for further study and research in brain surgery.

Dr. Mishra has inspired the organization of many groups in the United States and Canada who are studying Yoga Philosophy, Hatha Yoga and Self-Analysis in accordance with his teachings and under his direction.

This book has been compiled and illustrated by his student and a teacher of Hatha Yoga of New York, Goldie Lipson, artist.

OTHER ADDITIONS TO A YOGA PROGRAM

Dr. Rammurti Mishra has recommended other activities in his Yoga programs such as walking, dancing, all creative arts and crafts, music appreciation, singing, writing and listening to interesting and enlightening speakers.

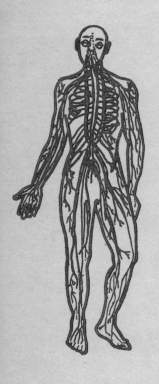

HOW TO USE THE HANDBOOK

The use of a mirror is helpful in many of the exercises and Asanas (Postures), in order to observe yourself in accordance with the illustrations.

The progressive arrangement of the lessons should help you in going from a simple exercise to more intricate advanced ones, as your body improves and becomes more flexible.

REJUVENATION

MENTAL-PHYSICAL-CONTROL

The eternal, youthful mind contains Mental Health through a physically healthy body. Such a mind seeks knowledge of Nature and Life, and is creative and imaginative.

ESSENCE OF "WHAT IS YOGA?"

Eight Steps

1. Yama — Control of the mind and mind waves.
2. Niyama — Observation of rules to obtain that aim.
3. Asanas — Postures.
4. Pranayama — Breathing exercises to help control of mind.
5. *Internal Instruments*
   Pratahara — Relaxation of organs and withdrawal of consciousness.
6. *Mental Analysis*
   Dharana — Fixation of consciousness on parts of anatomy or outside of body.
7. Dhyana — Constant suggestions.
8. Samadhi — Creation of will power and power of consciousness. Development of will power and intuition for the attainment of Supreme Consciousness. Samadhi depends on auto-suggestions. Manifestation of mental phenomena.

Four Systems

1. Hatha Yoga — Physical exercises.
2. Mantra Yoga — Psychological exercises and formulation of ideas.
3. Laya Yoga — Psychological application and absorption of mind stuff.
4. Raja Yoga — Identification with cosmic consciousness into ideas. The relation of physical and psychological exercises is interdependent — helping each other. Through mechanism of mental processes.

   A good body brings clear mental phenomena. There is identity of body and mind.

   Rigidity of mind and body is Death. Elasticity of mind and body is Life.

THE POWER OF SUGGESTION

Any knowledge that we are acquiring at present, in the past and that which we expect to acquire in the future will come to us through the power of suggestion.

Suggestion, concentration and daily practice are of utmost importance in obtaining that which is sought from Hatha Yoga.

Auto-suggestion is the greatest energy of all and is the greatest of all cures. By it, man can alleviate, minimize and eliminate fear of pain, torture, suffering, mental conflicts and, ultimately, all conflicts.

Its purpose is to gain control of mental and physical well being.

When a mental wave is projected from the subconscious mind it is called suggestion. If accepted in a form of an idea, image or an impulse of thought, it becomes a part of the conscious mind and part of individual personality.

All suggestions are auto-suggestions and are the greatest energy of all. It is the greatest of all cures. We are constantly moving by our suggestion.

RAJA YOGA

Yoga recognizes physics and metaphysics as one and is called Ultimate reality.

It is a science and study for mastery of mind and teaches how to conquer physical and mental weakness through philosophy, auto-suggestion, self-analysis, meditation and physical control (Hatha Yoga).

From Ignorance to Knowledge, from Darkness to Light, from Untruth to Truth, and from Unreality to Reality.

Yoga teaches the methods to control the mighty waves of the mind and to subdue them completely to the Primordial Consciousness which operates eternally through every perceptual mechanism. It is one of the six different approaches to the Wisdom teachings, leading to the Ultimate Truth.

Yoga is a collection of ancient disciplines, adopting numerous guises and techniques.

YOGANIDRA

Yoganidra is the state in which, through the Universal Magnetic Ocean of Consciousness, the entire body and senses are magnetized, through fixation, suggestion and sensation.

SAMPRA-SNATA SAMADHI

Sampra-Snata Samadhi is the state of Union of one's Individual Consciousness and Universal Consciousness, and Asam Prasnata Samadhi is the state of Absolute Individual Consciousness with Brahman Consciousness, Absolute Consciousness.

HATHA YOGA

Yoga is used to cure all physical and mental illness with absolute safety and without harm. It teaches spiritual, mental and physical control.

Yoga is a simple, easy to learn science, and like all sciences it is founded on facts.

Hatha Yoga trains the mind to sharpen the instruments of the body for the removal of the body's poisonous conditions; to remove fatigue and to arrest the tendency to decay and age. It is the science of gradual mastery of the body, through practice of physical and mental exercises and breath control. Every posture should give spiritual uplift and electromagnetic pulsation throughout the body. Hatha Yoga deals with various body positions and exercises through which alone the subtle machinery of the subconscious instincts can be controlled.

BENEFITS

1. Yama — Control of the mind and mental waves.
2. Niyama — Observation of rules to obtain that aim.
3. Asana — Different postures to obtain that state.
4. Pranayama — Regulation of breathing to help control of the mind.
5. Pratyahara — Complete relaxation of every organ and withdrawal of consciousness.
6. Dharana — Fixation of consciousness on different parts of the body.
7. Dhyana — Constant suggestions.
8. Samadhi — Creation of will power and power of consciousness.

Removes tension from body for chemical changes and mental therapy.

For more intense study of theory, methods and exercises on Raja Yoga, refer to Dr. Rammurti Mishra's book on "Fundamentals of Yoga," published by Julian Press.

HATHA — YOGA

Energy is Derived from All

DEFINITION = $\dfrac{\text{Ha—Moon}}{\text{Tha—Sun}}$ = Hatha

Name the twelve months of the year as
you assume the twelve positions.
Face the Sun.

For
Sunrise and Sunset

1
January
Om Mitraya
Namah

2
February
Om Navaya Namah
INHALE

3
March
Om Suryaya
Namah
EXHALE

4
April
Om Bhanave Namah
INHALE

5
May
Om Khagaya Namah
RETENTION OF BREATH

6
June
Om Pushe Namah
EXHALE

8-spots
TOUCH

7
July
Om Niranyagarbhaya
Namah
INHALE

Repeat same
on alternate leg.

8
August
Om Mareechaye
Namah
EXHALE

9
September
Om Savitre
Namah
INHALE

10
October
Om Arkaya
Namah
EXHALE

11
November
Om Aditaya
Namah
INHALE

12
December
Om
Bhaskaraya
Namah
EXHALE

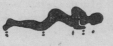

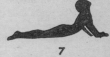

BENEFITS

Complete exercise for the stimulation of blood throughout body and joints.
Stretches muscles of entire body and joints.
A preventive and cure for all joint diseases.
Keeps body youthful, resilient and ageless.
The use of this exercise to start with will make it simpler for executing
all others.

ASANAS — POSTURES

DISCIPLINE OF THE BODY

The body and the mind are interdependent. The mind cannot function when the body is suffering from physical diseases, and the body is not normal when there are mental diseases. Yoga psychology recognizes the importance of both. It prescribes exercises for both the body and the mind so that they may develop in a psychophysiological equilibrium and so produce complete co-operation to manifest Universal Consciousness.

By meditation and practice of postures, consciousness becomes free from bondage and weakness and realizes a boundless existence of infinite bliss. Consciousness is manifested according to the development of the body and the mind; the body is the shadow of the mind.

MEDITATION

Dharana — Fixation.
Dhyana — Suggestion.
Samadhi — Concentration on flow of Consciousness.

TECHNIQUE:

Assume a relaxed position. Use any Asana (Pose) that is best for you. Adjust the mind by auto-suggestion to accept that which is Truth and beneficial and reject what is untruth and injurious.

BENEFITS:

Re-establishes confidence of the mind. Alleviates, minimizes and eliminates fear of pain, torture, suffering, mental conflicts, phobias and fear of death.

Helps remove any physical and mental disorder by auto-suggestion. Eventually with practicing relaxation of the entire body daily, we can attain perception of Supreme Consciousness.

(Read Dr. Mishra's books, "Fundamentals of Yoga," and "Yoga Psychology" for further study on this subject.)

ANAHAT NADAM — O M

O M is the Cosmic Vibration of the mind. It is the subtle and constant inexpressible musical vibration in the head. The humming sound is similar to the word Om. It is also manifested in many different divine sounds.

SUGGESTIONS

Believe in yourself and in your mind.

Nervous attitudes interfere with performance.

An unhappy and restless mind cannot concentrate.

Increase the atmosphere of expectancy and remove melancholy from the mind.

When a mental wave is projected from the subconscious mind, it is called suggestions. If accepted in a form of an idea, image or an impulse of thought, it becomes a part of the conscious mind and part of individual personality.

1. State of Mind — To think, reason and the like.

2. State of Speech — To form ideas.

3. State of Action — To form action.

3. State of Being — Being and Becoming.

For further study in these phases of Yoga refer to Raja Yoga, chapter two, three, and four in Dr. Rammurti Mishra's book, "Fundamentals of Yoga."

ASANAS — POSTURES

Use the same quiet, well venti-
lated room every day. At the
same time and before eating.
Wear comfortable clothes or
no clothes.

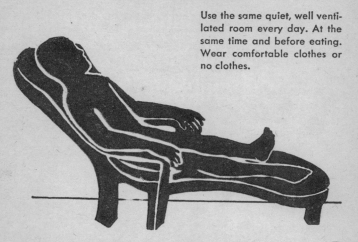

MEDITATION POSE — CONTOUR CHAIR

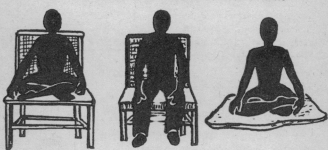

Lotus Pose   Chair Seat   Sukhasan—Easy Pose

Keep Head, Neck and Back always in a straight line.
Relax muscles, body and mind.
Breathe deeply, slowly and steadily.
Banish all extraneous thoughts.

Concentrate on **Relaxing** every external part of the body.
Start with the toes until you reach the top of head.
Continue by relaxing all internal organs.

ASANAS — POSTURES

SAVASANA

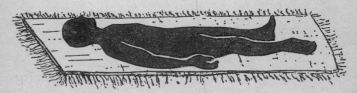

Relaxation — on mat.

Sun
Energy

WATER — SAVASANA

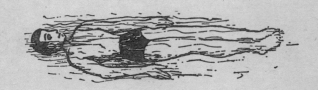

FLOATING ON THE WATER

Concentrate on **Relaxing** every external part of the body.
Start with the toes until you reach the top of head.
Continue by relaxing all internal organs.

Benefits:
    Brings tranquility and calmness.
    Restores vitality to muscles and internal organs.
    Equalizes blood circulation.
    Rejuvenates the entire body and mind.

ASANAS

Lotus Poses — Meditative Postures

Benefits: —Complete relaxation and equilibrium. Greater blood supply to pelvic region, benefiting coccygeal and sacral nerves. Enables one to contract and manipulate the abdominal muscles. Helps in acquiring electro-magnetic pulsation in the body and spiritual uplift.

SWASTIKASAN

Stretch Legs Wide & Forward

Lift Left Leg Flat against Right Thigh

Lift Right Leg over Left Leg

Keep Head, Neck and Back in a straight line.

PADMASAN

Stretch Legs

Put Right Foot over Left Thigh

Lift Left Foot on Right Thigh

Straighten Back. Keep Body erect

GUPTASAN

Stretch Legs (Used for Meditation)

Heel of Left Leg against Groin of Right Thigh

Lift Right Leg against Groin of Left Thigh

Keep Head, Neck & Back in a straight line.

SYMBOLIC MEDITATIVE POSE

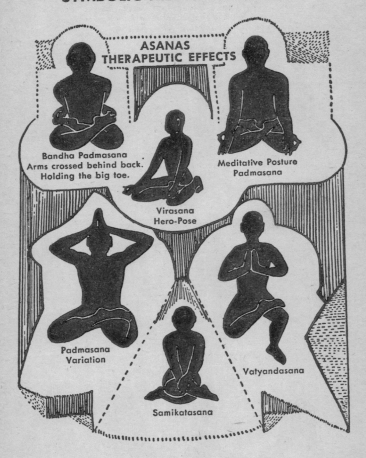

ASANAS
THERAPEUTIC EFFECTS

Bandha Padmasana
Arms crossed behind back.
Holding the big toe.

Virasana
Hero-Pose

Meditative Posture
Padmasana

Padmasana
Variation

Samikatasana

Vatyandasana

ASANAS — POSTURES

SYMBOLIC MEDITATIVE POSES

SUKHASANA — EASY POSE

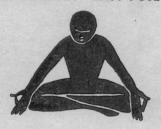

O M POSE

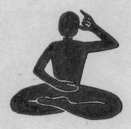

SIDDHASANA — The Perfect Pose

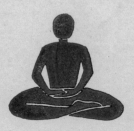

SALUTATION TO THE SUPREME

BEGINNERS

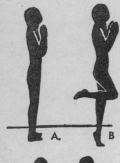

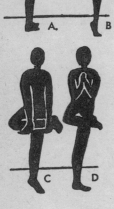

Technique:

A — Stand erect with palms together in front of chest.

B — Raise one foot up and back with knee bent.
Slowly rise on toes and hold this pose.
Before you begin to lose balance rest with both feet on the ground.

C — With both hands, bring Leg up and across the thigh of the opposite Leg.

D — Bring palms together in front of chest.

ADVANCED

E — Slowly rise on toes. Hold this position as long as you can.

F — Raise arms bringing palms together over head.

Benefits:

Rejuvenates the entire central nervous system and the peripheral nervous system.
Control of balance.

Experience:

Will result in the quivering of the nerves from the soles of the foot you are standing on to the top of the nerve centers.

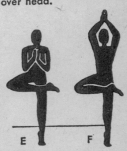

LORD MATARAJASAN POSE AND VARIATIONS

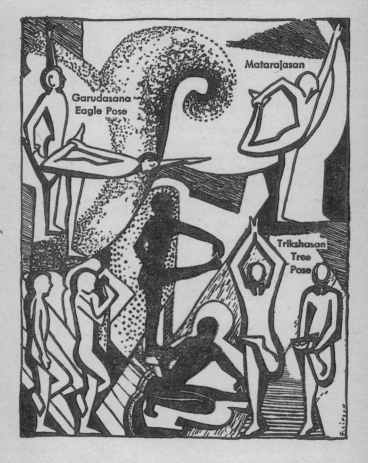

PRANA AND PRANAYAMA

1. PRANA — Force of motion, magnetism, gravitation, electricity, wound, wind, heat, thought, etc., are examples of Prana.
The sum total of all forces in the Universe, mental and physical, when resolved back to the original state is called Prana.
Prana is expanded by thinking, willing, acting, moving, talking, writing, etc.

2. PRANAYAMA — Control of Universal Prana.
Breathing exercise is one of the many exercises through which one arrives at real Pranayama. Concentration, meditation and study of Self-analysis is Pranayama.

3. PURAKAM — Inhalation. Filling lungs and cells with fresh air.

4. KUMBHAKAM — Retention. Restraining of air.
Exchange of gaseous substance. Toxic air is replaced by fresh primal energy in the tissues and lungs.

5. RECAKAM — Exhalation.
All toxic air and other toxic substances are removed from the chest.

BREATHING EXERCISES

Biological life and consciousness depends on breathing.
Breathing consists of three states:

1. INHALATION — The filling of one's lungs and cells with air. (Purakam)

2. RETENTION — The state of restraining the air. An exchange of gaseous substance, toxic air with fresh Prana in the tissues and lungs.

3. EXHALATION — By this process all the toxic air and other toxic substances are removed by the lungs. The atmospheric pressure separates forcefully on the whole body to stimulate every body tissue. (Recakam)

PRANA AND PRANAYAMA

CONTROL OF RESPIRATION

Through breathing exercises, we strengthen both respirations directly.

Internal and external pressure comes into friction and consequently they awaken the entire central nervous system, and the senses.

Internal Respiration consists of *Metabolic* actions and reactions.

With every inspiration in succession, Universal energy, life and light of knowledge are drawn into the body through the lungs and skin which are the main systems of respiration.

With every expiration in succession, impurities of the body are removed through the lungs, skin and kidneys.

One should do breathing exercises up to the point of exhaustion and perspiration; these are the signs of internal respiration. When perspiration and exhaustion start, one should stop the breathing exercises at this point to give internal respiration a chance to operate fully.

Energy of the sun operates freely in the body through conduction, convection and radiation. The inner light continually increases until it reaches full freedom or salvation.

The body tissues, especially nerve tissues, cannot live without oxygen and oxygen is part of Prana which we breathe with inspiration.

PRANAYAMA

DEEP BREATHING EXERCISES

"That state in which the respiratory system is trained by forcing air in and out is called the breathing exercise of Pranayama."

Just as a vacuum cleaner removes all kinds of dirt from the house, so the suction machine of breathing exercises sucks up all defects from the body, senses and mind. Then removing them through expiration, perspiration and other excretory channels.

The body and nerve tissues receive oxygen in every act of breathing and with the added stimulant of all exercises this is increased.

PRANAYAMA

DEEP BREATHING EXERCISES

Start these exercises slowly, increasing the speed gradually until you do them as rapidly as possible.

When completely exhausted, stop and relax.

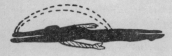

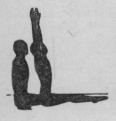

Inhale as you stretch and raise hands over head. Exhale as you lower arms.

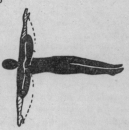

Inhale as you extend arms out. Exhale as hands are placed on diaphragm.

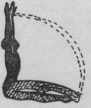

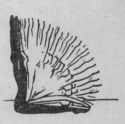

Inhale as you stretch and raise hands over head. Exhale as you lower arms. Keep legs straight. Back and arms stretching as you bend up and down at the waist. Start slowly, reaching up as high as possible, and touching toes as you exhale on going down.

Start this exercise slowly, increasing the speed gradually until you do them as rapidly as possible. When completely exhausted, stop and relax.

HATHA YOGA — PRANAYAMA EXERCISES

Traditional method of closing the nostrils for *Alternate* breathing—
Anuloma Viloma Pranayama.

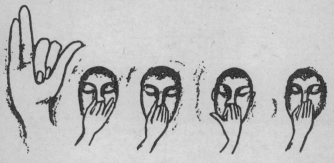

Use right hand. Inhale   Close   Exhale   Close

TECHNIQUE: — Assume a relaxed position.

1. Press right thumb to right nostril — Inhale through the left nostril.
2. Press pinky and ring finger to left nostril — Retention of breath.
3. Release right thumb — Exhale through the right nostril.
4. Close the right nostril again with the thumb — Hold.
5. Open the left nostril — Inhale — Close both nostrils. Repeat again from #1.

YOGAMUNDRA   BREATH CONTROL

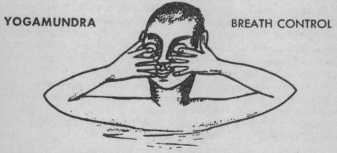

Listening to Nadam (om sound) by artificial Mudra technique and seeing the spectrum of lights.

Fill mouth with air and close eyes, nostrils, ears and press lips together. Hold Breath.

WATER PRANAYAMA

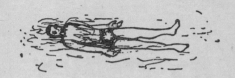

FLOATING

Relaxing completely. Inhale through nose or mouth. Exhale slowly through nose. Concentrate on relaxing every part of external body from toes to top of head.

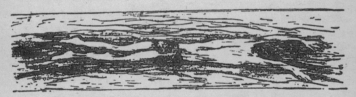

Floating completely relaxed. Exhaling slowly.

PRANAYAMA BENEFITS

By counter-reacting on inspiration and expiration, both movements are kept in check and the respiratory center in the medulla comes under control. This leads to the subjugation of the senses and mind; increases strength and energy; sharpens the intellect; develops the hormonal secretions and vital forces in the human body; thus producing courage and control of the senses.

Awakens entire central nervous system. Produces purification and firmness of the mind senses and consciousness. Life is manifested in its true form for checking the restless mind.

For further study of Pranayama, refer to Chapter 25, in "Fundamentals of Yoga" by Dr. Mishra.

PRANA — PRANAYAMA EXERCISES

Pranayama, before meditation, helps the mind to become one-pointed. Done vigorously, it becomes a powerful exercise for various internal organs and the whole body.

BAHYA VRITTI

External forceful location of physiological and psychic energy and Prana.

1. Forcibly throw out the air through the nose and mouth.
2. Inhale and check the breath as long as possible.
3. Before expelling the breath, the pelvis should be pulled upward and kept up as long as the breath remains out.
4. When there is a feeling of uneasiness and suffocation, the breath should be slowly drawn in.
5. Repeat according to the capacity and desire.
6. Relax mentally by listening to the OM sound. The OM sound is the ringing or any sound heard in the head or ears.

ABHYANTATA VRITTI — INTERNAL PRANAYAMA

The first Pranayama ends in the second.

1. Inhale and hold the breath as long as possible.
2. Exhale and hold breath. Inhale and hold. Keep this up to capacity. This makes one cycle of Pranayama.

STUMBHA VRITTI — MOTIONLESS PRANAYAMA

1. Air is neither taken in nor removed.
2. It is immediate checking and stopping of air all at once; inside and outside.
3. The chest remains like a straight pillar in a standstill position or motionless jar full of liquid.

BAHYA BHYANATA — OUT-IN-HOLDING PRANAYAMA

1. Draw air in deeply through the nose and hold.
2. When the tendency is to exhale — forcibly breathe in another amount of air through the nose.
3. Exhale and remove all air from chest. Hold and keep exhaling alternately as long as possible.

KAPALA — ABDOMINAL MOVEMENTS

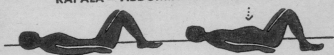

TECHNIQUE:
Take a relaxed position with knees up and feet almost together. Exhale completely through the nose. Feel the spine touching the ground. Abdomen becomes concave. Slowly inhale through nose. Concentrate on sending the air to chest diaphragm and stomach. Hold air as long as comfortable. Exhale slowly. Relax then repeat.

BENEFITS: — This simple breathing exercise relieves tensions, relaxes body and mind. Quiets nerves.

UDDIYANA BANDHA — PELVIC CONTRACTION

| Madhyama (Central Nauli) | | Uttar (Left side Nauli) | Dakshina (Right — Nauli) |

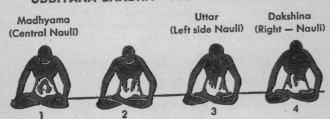

TECHNIQUE:

1. Exhale Completely. Bend head-shoulders slightly forward to deepest exhalation. Abdomen becomes concave. Chest expands. Hold a few seconds. Relax abdomen and inhale.

2. During expiratory breath suspension, in #1, try to cause the rectus abdominis to stand out against the collapsed abdomen by pressing hands against thighs and making a forward-downward abdominal thrust. Concentrate on this procedure. Control the isolated rectus abdominis for a few seconds. Inhale slowly. Relax.

3. When control of central position is accomplished, shifting to left and right is just more concentrated control.

4. Do not overdo these exercises at first efforts. These should be done slowly and gradually.

BENEFITS: — The entire abdominal region and internal organs obtain marvelous health results. The advanced stages of Vajroli (suction) which follows, is best obtained through instruction from a Yogi Teacher.

KAPALA IN LOTUS POSITION
ABDOMINAL MOVEMENTS

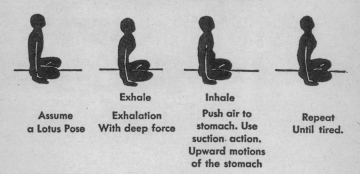

	Exhale	Inhale	
Assume a Lotus Pose	**Exhalation With deep force**	**Push air to stomach. Use suction action. Upward motions of the stomach**	**Repeat Until tired.**

CONCENTRATE: — On stomach, colon, intestines, liver, kidneys, gall bladder, pancreas and reproductive organs and glands.

BENEFITS: — Reach all these parts.

KAPALA BHATI — BLACKSMITH BELLOWS
ALSO CALLED
BHASTRIKA — BELLOWS IN SANSKRIT

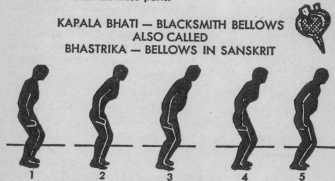

1   2   3   4   5

1. Hands on knees (or hips). Knees slightly bent.
2. Exhale with force.
3. Begin inhalation and exhalation—quickly and rhythmically. Resembling a pair of Blacksmith Bellows.

BENEFITS: — The Benefits mentioned in above Kapala also apply to Blacksmith Bellows. Because of extra force used, the nerves and blood circulation receive extra benefits from toes to the head. Stimulates metabolism. Prevents constipation. Firms and strengthens the abdomen. Beneficial to the organs and glands of the Viscera.

BHALASPRESTRESLANJANU

MERUDANDASANA
VARIATION OF
PAVANAMKTASANA

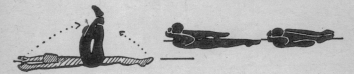

JELY-FISH-FLOAT

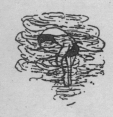

— (Holding breath under water.)
Similar benefits as above.
Relax completely—Take a *small* amount
of air through nose. Bend at waist—
Head to knees—Arms around legs. Hold
this position until you feel the need of
air. As you raise your head — Breathe
out gently.

Embryo Float

Bring knees to head
very slowly.

Jelly Fish Float

Slowly bend at waist
by reaching down
and clasp ankles.

Stretching Legs slowly

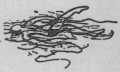

Point Toes.

PAVANAMUKTASANA — Head to Knee

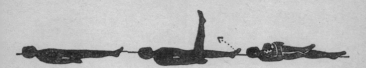

Inhale — Slowly raise leg parallel to body. Exhale — Press knee, with hands to chest.

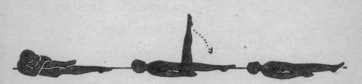

Raise head to knee. Inhale — Slowly lay head back — Raise leg — Exhale — Lower leg slowly. Alternate leg — Concentrate on slow stretching movements and Pressing down the Knee.

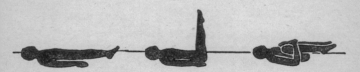

Inhale — Slowly raise both legs. Exhale — Press both legs to chest.

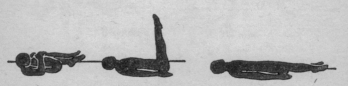

Retention of breath. Raise head to knees. Inhale — Exhale — As you slowly lower legs.

JANU SIRASANA — Head to Knee Poses

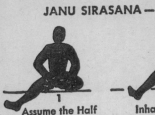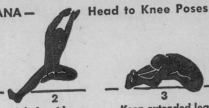

1
Assume the Half Lotus. Put the sole of one foot high up and flat against the thigh of the opposite leg.

2
Inhale with arms overhead. Exhale as you reach down and out to touch toes. Hold down position.

3
Keep extended leg straight. Hold pose, with natural breathing. Alternate sides. Hold Big Toe.

With Both Legs Forward

JANU SIRASANA
BHUNAMAN ASANA — Forward Head Bend
HASTHA PADASON

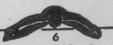

4
Stretch legs straight out. Inhale.

5
Exhale as you bend at waist and clasp feet or toes.

6
When possible—Put chin or forehead to floor. Use natural breathing and hold a short time.

BENEFITS: — Concentration is on the hamstring muscles, legs, arms, spine, hip joints, abdominal muscles. The pelvic and perineal parts are being used.

KARMASAN — Tortoise Pose

PRANATASANA
Forward Reach

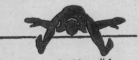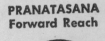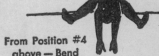

From Position #4 above — Bend forward and bring arms under knees. Hold.

From Position #4 above — Bend forward and down, until trunk, head and arms touch the ground.

BENEFITS: — The same benefits as for Janu Sirasana, above, with extra stretch used.

32

HALASANA — Plough Pose

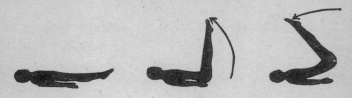

Relax. Inhale deeply.   Exhale slowly as you raise legs

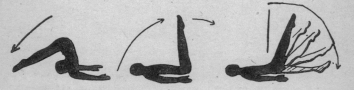

straight up and over.   Exhale slowly as you *lower back* and legs.
Hold Plough Pose.
Breathe slowly.

Concentrate on the Vertebral Column
pressing on the ground from the neck
to the top of the spine.

BENEFITS: — Removes joint diseases. Reduces abdominal and chest fat, as it
stretches the muscles. Renders the
spine elastic and supple. Stimulates
the thyroid, hormones and health of
the entire body. Develops a straight
back and active muscles. Relieves
constipation.

VARIATIONS OF HALASANA — Plough Pose

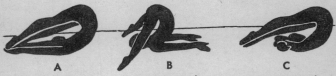

A	B	C
Toes to Fingers.	Legs Spread.	Arms Crossed.

A — Hold toes with hands. This variation puts pressure on the lower part of the spine.

B — Spread legs with short steps to sides of shoulders.

C — Arms crossed behind shoulders.

Breathe slowly through the nose. Concentrate or Meditate. Keep legs straight with toes pointed throughout Asanas-(Poses).

BENEFITS: — Removes joint diseases. Reduces abdominal and chest fat, as it stretches the muscles. Renders the spine elastic and supple. Stimulates the thyroid, hormones and health of the entire body. Develops a straight back and active muscles. Relieves constipation.

HALASAN — Plough Posture

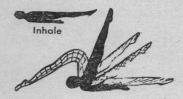

Inhale

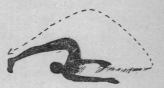

Exhale

Lie flat on back, palms down, arms at sides, slowly raise hips and without bending knees bring legs overhead until toes touch ground.

Hold Pose
Natural Breathing.

Touch Toes to Hands.

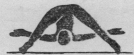

Spread Legs.

Knees to Shoulders

Advanced

Balancing
on upper part of back.

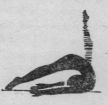

Advanced Halasan.

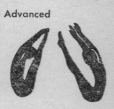

Balancing
on the buttocks

BENEFITS: — Reduces abdominal and chest fat. Keeps the spine elastic. Strengthens muscles of abdomen, legs and back and flexibility of the spine. Stimulates thyroid and all the vertebra and ligaments of the cervical region. Improves the posture.

SUPTA VAJRASAN — VARIATIONS
Natasira   Chakrasana — Wheel Pose

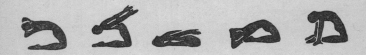

Take kneeling pose. Bending slowly back take different positions. Hold them.

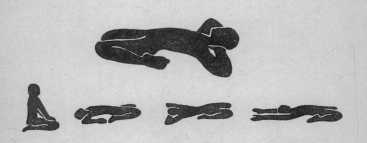

1. Kneel with heels touching body-toes pointing out. Lean slowly back putting weight on elbows and buttocks.

2. Slowly lower back and shoulders to ground. Bring arms in back of head —

3. or stretched back over head. To regain kneeling position put arms back to the sides of body. Bend forward.

BENEFITS: — (For above Asanas—Positions) Gives flexibility to the back, legs, toes and spine. Develops chest and bust. Relieves tension through spine and neck. Abdominal recti, pelvic region and sexual organs are benefited.

PASCHIMATANASANA — Head to Knee Pose

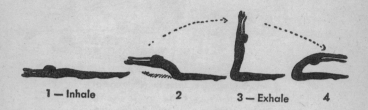

1 — Inhale   2   3 — Exhale   4

Lie flat on your back. Arms overhead.
Keeping legs firmly on the floor, stiffen
body and slowly raise head and chest to
position #3. Reaching up — down and
out.

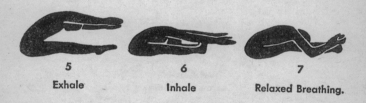

5   6   7
Exhale   Inhale   Relaxed Breathing.

Reaching out to and beyond toes. Hold
toes and position. Head is on knees.

BENEFITS: — Stimulation for abdominal
viscera as kidneys, liver, and pancreas. Spine, legs, hamstring muscles
and neck are strengthened.

VARIATIONS OF ADVANCED HALASANA
Plough Posture

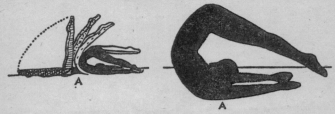

A — Gradually lengthen the distance of toes from your head by stretching slowly. It is not wise to hasten this. Avoid straining.

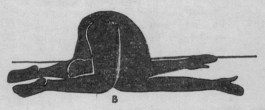

B — Bring knees to shoulders. Press legs against ears.

VARIATION
As an Exercise.

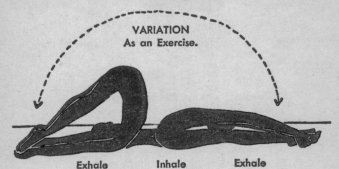

Exhale   Inhale   Exhale

BENEFITS:— Increases the benefits of the Plough Posture. Eliminates excess fat from abdomen. Tones up the spine and central nervous system.

KAPATHASA — Pigeon Pose

  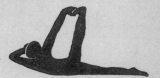

Bend knee — Put foot on sole of left thigh.

Pull left leg with both hands — Touch back of head.

Hand to Toe Pull.

JANU SIRASAN — Variation

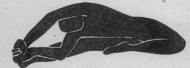 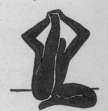

One leg is stretched sideward. Foot of the other leg is bent with the sole on the outstretched leg. This foot is brought up on the thigh as is comfortable. Bend to side and clasp outstretched foot with both hands. Body held to side — All in a straight line.

From Lotus pose — Bring leg straight up. Hold and balance.

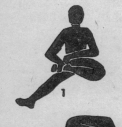
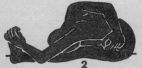

Put foot on thigh — puts pressure on abdominal viscera when spine is bent. Head is on knee — Grab toe from behind back.

Asanas on this page:—

BENEFITS:—Concentrate on spine, head and hamstrings.

Note: — Inhale in upright positions and Exhale in down ones. (All)

39

ASANAS
YOGA MUDRA — Spiritual Attitude

Meditate in all these Asanas.

Mind is controlling
to give beneficial results.

Kneeling
position.

Bend Head in
clasped hands.

Head on folded
arms.
Arms on knees.

Lotus Pose. Clasp
hands in back.
Put head to
ground.
Raise arms up.

MANDUSKANA — Frog Pose
Back Views

Kneel with legs
to the sides.

Heels together.

Press knees to
ground with the
palms of hands.

GOMUKHASANA
Cow Head

Kneel with legs on the side.
Clasp hands behind back
— one arm over the shoul-
der — other arm from
across back.

BANDHA PADMASAN
Bound Lotus Pose

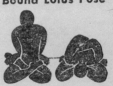

Take the Lotus Pose. Cross
arms in back. Catch toes
with hands. Bend head to
ground.

MATSYASANA — Fish Pose

Beginners

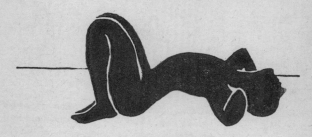

Hands behind neck. Heels against buttocks—knees bent. Arch upper back with head as far back as possible. Hold position.

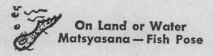 On Land or Water
Matsyasana — Fish Pose

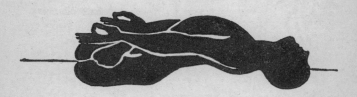

Take the Lotus pose on back. Hold feet or toes. Slowly bend back, lifting knees vertically. When back is on ground, lower knees and arch the spine. Bring head back as far as possible. The weight is on buttocks, vertex and crown of Head.

BENEFITS: — Stretches neck, spinal and back muscles.

AKRANA DHANURASA — Bow Shooting Pose

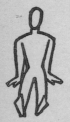

Sit with
legs extended.

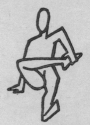

Grasp ankle and
draw leg across
and back of
body.
Use hand of
opposite side.
Press back and
hold pose.

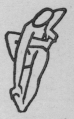

Lean forward
and hold foot
of the
extended leg.
Press back
and hold.

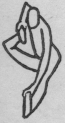

Use the hand
of the same side.
Draw one leg
back at the
same time
hold foot
extended.

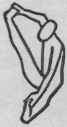

Straighten
the back leg
and keep
extended leg
out.

Alternate all poses.

BENEFITS: — Stimulates abdominal muscles, spine and neck. Keeps muscles
of legs and thighs elastic and strong.
Stretches hamstring muscles and
makes hip joints flexible.

ELKA PADA SIRASAN — Leg and Head Pose

These are advanced Asanas — advance slowly.

Leg and Head Pose

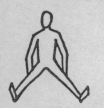 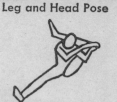 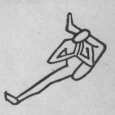

Pull foot directly above head and back of neck.
Bring palms together in front of head.

OM Pose

Leg & Head Pose

OMKARASANA-PRANAVASANA

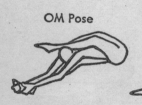 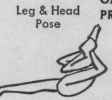

OM Pose
Bend forward
and clasp ankle
or foot
with both hands.

Leg & Head Pose
Bring one leg
in back of neck
and across
both shoulders.
Hold ankle
with both hands.

Bring
outstretched leg
up into the
space between
the side of
the body
and the thigh.

YOGA DANTA ASANA

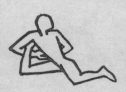

Spread legs
very wide apart.
Bring one leg
straight up behind the
shoulder of the same
side. Turn head to the
opposite side.

BENEFITS: — Stimulates abdominal muscles, spine and neck. Keeps muscles
of legs and thighs elastic and strong.
Stretches hamstring muscles and
makes hip joints flexible.

HIP — LEG STRETCH

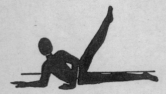

Inhale — Retain
Up

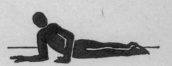

Exhale — Inhale
Together

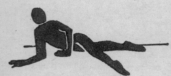

Exhale — Hold
Front

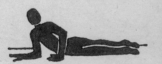

Inhale
Together

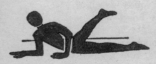

Retain — (Back)

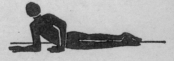

Exhale — Relax

Turn to the other side and repeat.

BENEFITS: — Streamlines hips, legs and
waist line.

ASANA

Parsva Bhunaman   Natasirasana   Pranatasana

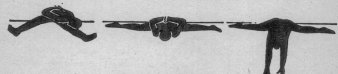

Alternate sides.

Legs spread wide.
Hands clasped behind.

Stretch arms forward.

Exhale as you bend forward in these three Asanas. Slowly bend outward, forward and then down until head touches the farthest point of contact. Do not bend the knees.

STAMBHASANA — Pillar Pose

Pelvic Exercise

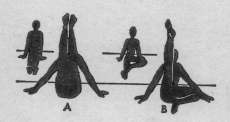

A   B

TECHNIQUE

A — Arms are parallel to hips.
Keeping legs stiff, raise legs as far back toward the body as possible. Hold—then slowly lower legs.

B — From half Lotus Pose, slowly raise leg as described above.

BENEFITS: — Stretches limbs and torso.

ADVANCED ASANAS

Omkarasana Pose

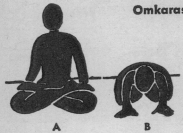

A — From Lotus posture —
Slowly raise body and
B — rest on knees and hands.

A   **B**

Pasini Mudra

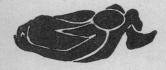

Next, pull left foot over head
and over right foot. Interlock
the fingers at the hip joint.
Concentrate on pelvic and
perineal area.

Parvatasana —
Mountain Posture

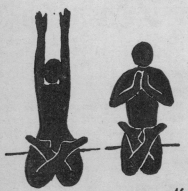

From Lotus pose — Slowly
raise both arms upward as
you balance on knees.

Leg Stretching Exercises

Beginners and Advanced

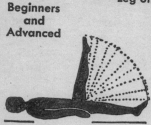

Inhale before lifting legs. Exhale as legs are slowly lowered. Keep legs straight. point toes.

Arms are at the sides. Palms flat on the ground.

Left Leg

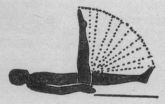

Alternate legs.

Right Leg

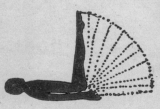

Raise both legs up perpendicular, to body and slowly lower. Legs kept straight.

BENEFITS: — Pelvic region and legs are stretched and stimulated by both exercises; reduces fat from hips, stomach and thighs.

Both Legs

LEG STRETCHING EXERCISES

Lying on back, Arms are at shoulder level. Palms flat on the ground.

Inhale

Exhale

Slow Swing Across

Inhale

Return to Original

Relax
Inhale and Repeat cycle
with alternate leg.

Inhale

Draw up
and across

Inhale

Exhale

Relax

Inhale and Repeat cycle starting from the alternate side.

BENEFITS: — Reduces flabbiness of hips and waist line.

SARVANGASANA — Shoulder Stand

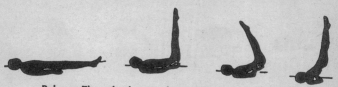

Relax — Then slowly raise legs and hips straight up.

Use hands and arms to support the back.
Move hands up until you reach the shoulders.
The weight of the body is on the upper back of
the neck and across the top of the shoulders.
Legs are perpendicular to the body.

LOWERING THE BODY

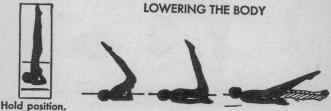

Hold position.

In lowering the body, arms are brought to the sides. Weight of
body is on the arms. Legs are slowly brought down until hips are
resting on the ground.

Increase the length of time you hold this position gradually. The
breathing should be natural. Concentrate on the circulation of
blood through the body.

TIME: — From one to fifteen minutes.

BENEFITS: — The stomach muscles are being used in lowering the
legs. Stretches the spine. Relaxes the legs and other areas
through relief of pressure. In some cases removes enlargements
of veins of the legs. Improves the general metabolism.

Stimulates thyroid hormones and improves health. Rejuvenates
entire body and sex glands of both sexes. Beneficial for displaced
uterus, etc. Prevents accumulation of fat on abdomen. Improves the
blood circulation.

CHILDREN: — This Asana will stimulate growth in children and improve intelligence and memory. It should be done at least once
a day.

THE KING OF ALL ASANÀS
SIRS.HASANA — Head Stand

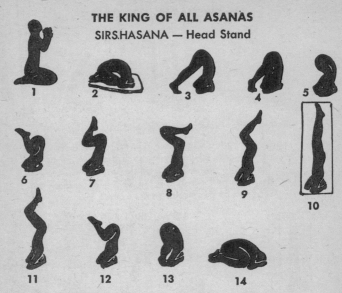

1. Kneel with heels and knees together. Sit back on heels.
2. Elbows and interlocked fingers form a triangle on ground. Place back of head in cupped hands, close to knees. Elbows are close to the sides of knees which will be about a foot apart for balance. The _top_ of head, near the forehead, rests on protected ground.
3. The weight of body will be supported on elbows, arms and locked fingers. Arch back. Rise on toes to test balance and support.
4. Walk forward until knees are close to body.
5. When trunk is comfortably arched.
6. Raise legs with knees bent.
7. Slowly and hold next position.
8. Movements are done very slowly while concentrating on the fact that your weight is on your arms as you reach up with your legs.
9. In this completed position, relax the whole body.
10. This position is held for a minute at the beginning, increasing gradually to fifteen or twenty minutes. Some Yogis like to keep this position longer.

LOWERING THE BODY

11, 12, 13. Lower legs very slowly. Feel that you are tucking your knees under to your chest.
14. Hold last position a few minutes as the blood circulation harmonizes.

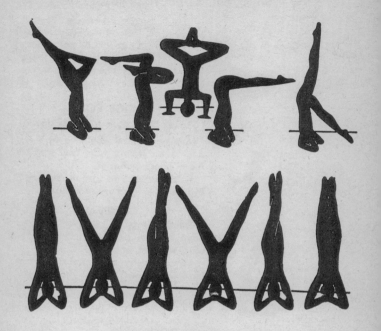

SIRSASANA LEG EXERCISE

Assume the Head Stand position. Spread —
Cross — Spread — Cross Legs.

BENEFITS: — for Sirsasana (Head Stand) and
Variations. Sends increased blood supply to
brain, pineal body and pituitary gland.
Benefits cardiac and digestive systems, liver,
spleen and sexual regeneration. Relieves
asthmatic discomfort, headaches, dizziness
and arterio-sclerosis. Treats the degenera-
tion of nerve centers and tones up the
nervous system. Improves intelligence and
memory.

SARVANGASANA VARIATIONS

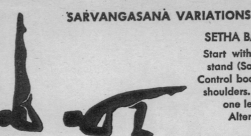

SETHA BANDHASAN

Start with the shoulder stand (Sarvangasana). Control body on arms and shoulders. Slowly lower one leg to floor. Alternate leg.

BRIDGE POSE

Lower other leg to form a bridge.

Another method would be from rest position on ground, raise back with the aid of hands and arms.

Hold position for a comfortable length of time using regular breathing.

VIPARETA

Follow directions given on previous page for the Head-Stand (Saravangasana) stopping at position 4.

Concentrate on pointing toes, straight legs, weight on the arms, upper back and the back of the neck. Natural breathing.

SARVANGASANO

This Asana is described on previous page.

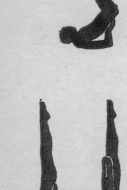

When you attain perfection in this with the arms holding the weight of the body and the hands on upper back, shift weight of body back to neck and back of head. This naturally brings the chin to the chest. Remove the hands from the back and very slowly slide them along the thighs until they are close and straight at the sides of the body.

Gradually increase the length of time you hold this position. Concentrate on keeping the body upright in a straight line from back of neck to toes. Judge this by the angle of hips, knees and toes as you see them from your position.

OORDHWAPADMASAN
Head stand — Lotus pose — Side bend

TECHNIQUE: — From Head Stand very slowly bend left leg — Place foot on right thigh — Right leg over left thigh. Bend slowly at waist. Hold. Alternate side.

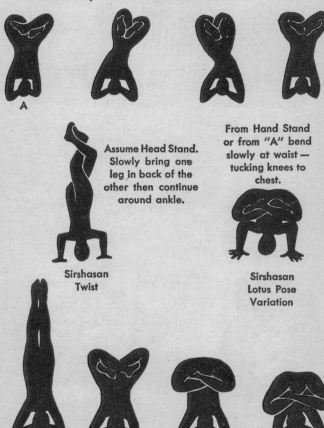

A

Assume Head Stand. Slowly bring one leg in back of the other then continue around ankle.

Sirshasan Twist

From Hand Stand or from "A" bend slowly at waist — tucking knees to chest.

Sirshasan Lotus Pose Variation

Urdhva Pudmasana

Oordhwapadmasan

Shyam Sunda

Goswami

ADVANCED ASANAS

UTTIDA PADMASAN

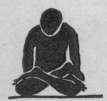

Rock back and forth.

KURMASANA —
Half Tortoise Posture
Beginners Swing.

From kneeling position with palms on ground, raise the body on the balanced hands. Rock body back and forth in a swinging motion.

KUKUTASAN —
Cock Posture

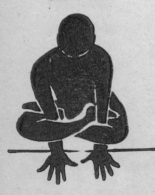

From Uttida Padmasan Pose put hands through legs — Palms on ground—Raise body.

UTTHITA SAMAKONSANA

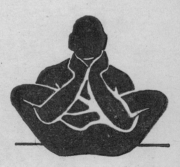

From Uttida Padmasan insert arms through legs—Put hands at neck.

From kneeling position—Raise body on the balanced hands. Rock body back and forth in a swinging motion.

FOR ADVANCED STUDENTS

LOLASAN — Mayoorasan Pose

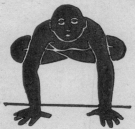

Assume Lotus Pose Uttida Padmasan.
Hands and forearms are firm and steady
to support body. Raise up slowly.

UTTIDA PADMASAN

UTHITHA KURMASAN — Tortoise Pose

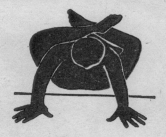

Place right foot behind Head — Wedged
against nap of neck — Left foot behind
right in an Ankle lock. Balance on hands.

BENEFITS: — Increases breathing capacity. Stomach, liver, pancreas, kidneys,
valar and dorsal carpal ligaments at
waist, and arms all benefit.

VRISCHIKASAN — Scorpion Pose

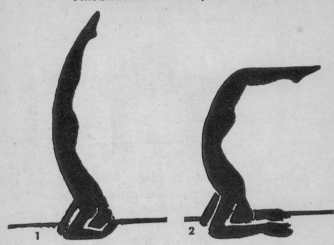

1. From Sirshasan (Head Stand) Bend knees.

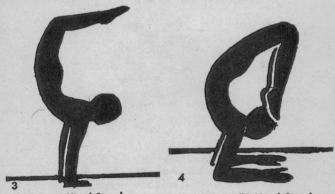

3. From Hand Stand —
Bend knees.

4. From #1 Head Stand —
raise head to meet feet.

2—3—4 — When bending legs do this
very slowly. For lowering body — see
chapter for "Head Stand."

SIRSHASANA — Head Stand Variations
ADVANCED POSES

One Hand Stand —
On Ball

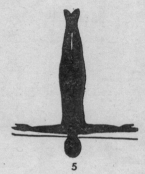

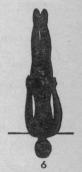

6
6. After #5

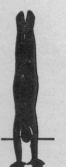

9

5

5. Do head stand with hands flat on the ground instead of clasped on back of head. Remove hands slowly out to the sides.

9. From #8 — Bend body to side — Then raise arm.

7. From Hand stand #8 — Bring one leg down to head by bending at the knee. Alternate to other leg.

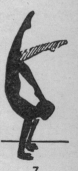

8

7

BENEFITS: — Spiritual and mental powers. All benefits are similar to Head Stand (Sirshasana.)

BHUYJANGOSAN — Cobra Pose

ASANA

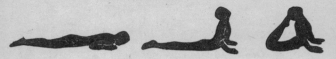

Palms level at shoulders.
Inhale.
Repeat slowly.

Do not raise hips from ground.
Retention of breath.
Hold pose a little longer each time.

COBRA EXERCISE

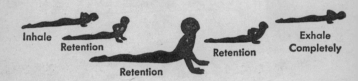

Inhale

Retention

Retention

Retention

Exhale
Completely

Do not raise hips from ground.

Start exercise slowly — Then gradually increase speed until you are exhausted.

BENEFITS: — Excellent for increasing capacity of lung power, breath control.

This is one of the best breathing exercises. Very simple to do, yet the most beneficial for all ages and all health conditions.

Stimulates the blood and energy to glands, chest, neck, spine and brain. Heart and lung muscles are strengthened.

ARHDA SALABHASA — Half Locust

LEG AND BACK STRETCH

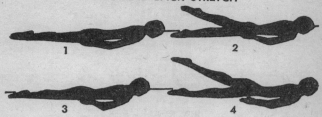

1. Inhale. 2. Slowly raise leg. Hold. 3. Exhale and slowly lower leg. 4. Inhale — Repeat — Alternate legs. Use fists under hip bones for assistance in raising body up. The chin is on the ground. Keep knees straight — Stretch leg and toes pointed out and up.

LOCUST

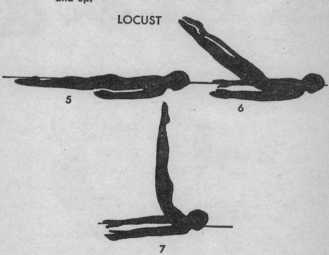

5.-6. Inhale and slowly raise both legs.
7. Advanced Locust position.

BENEFITS: — Tones up muscles of the entire body and glands. All limbs, spine and stomach muscles are stretched and stimulated by this exercise.

59

PASCHIMOTTANASEN — Forward and Back Roll

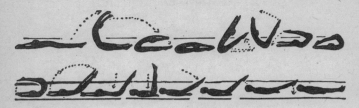

ROCK AND ROLL

Exercise

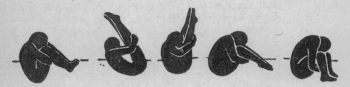

VARIATIONS

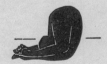

KARNA PEEDASAN —
Closed Plough Pose

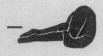

KARNA PEEDASAN —
Ear Knee — Pose

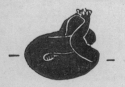

VARIATIONS

HALASAN — Plough Posture

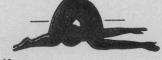

ASANAS

CATOKASANA —
Cuckoo Pose

Bridge

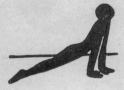
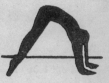

MAKARASANA —
Cobra

SARPASANA —
Snake Posture

BHUJANGENDRASAN —
King Cobra

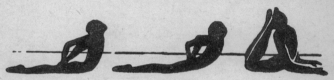

In all the above Asanas, Inhale and keep retention of air in the Posture pose. Exhale then relax. The length of time one holds the position will increase with practice.

Concentrate on working the spinal and back muscles.

When these poses are accomplished with ease, Inhale — retain air as long as comfortable, then release air slowly. Rest.

BENEFITS:— The Head, neck, spine, trunk, hips, thighs, legs, toes and especially the dorsolumbar region receive great benefits from these Asanas.

ASANAS

DOLASANA — Swing Posture

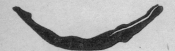

NAUKASANA — Boat Pose

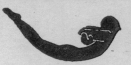

Stretch body. Inhale and Exhale as you swing both legs up and down. This can be done at the same time or rock back and forth. First raise your head—lower head as you raise your legs. Repeat slowly until you are rocking forward and back.

Can be done the same as the Swing Posture but the fact that the arms are crossed behind the back makes this more difficult.

From the Diving Board

By extending the body partly off the board (just beyond the chest) you roll fast and throw the legs over and back. (Locust Technique) Keep hands locked or together until you are ready to come up.

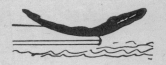

BENEFITS: — Massages all parts of the body as you rock. Improves circulation and promotes physical well-being.

Basic — MATSYASANA — The Fish

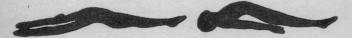

Stretch — inhale as you lift chest up. In two positions.

BENEFITS: — Complete stretching exercise. Good for reducing stomach fat.

MAYURASANA — Peacock Pose

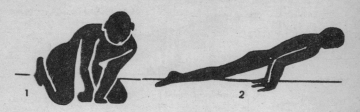

1. Kneel on ground with palms of hands flat down between knees. Test your balance by rising on your toes. Fingers facing towards you
2. Straighten body with the toes touching ground. Raise hips above elbows.

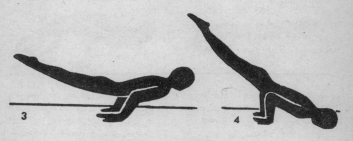

3. Resting hips on elbows — Slowly raise legs until they are straight out in back
4. Place forehead on the ground and raise body in a straight line

BENEFITS: — Elbow pressing into abdomen and liver increases the blood supply. Relieves chest and abdominal diseases. Reduces abdominal fat, piles and constipation. Helps evacuation of excretory system Helps balance the body

ONE ARM PEACOCK POSE

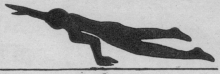

5

5. Assume position #1 with palm directly in front of you — Fingers towards you — Bend forward — Place abdomen on the same elbow and extend body forward — Legs backward — Balance will be on the elevated elbow — Legs apart — Extend arm — Maintain the final attitude for a time. Alternate to other arm

LOLASANA

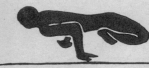

6

6. From Lotus Pose — Stand on knees (Parvatasana — Mountain Posture) Then lean forward — place the palms in front of you on the ground — Fingers towards you — Forearms vertical and close enough for good balance. Bend forward — Abdomen on elbow joints and balance body as in illustration #3.

EKAHASTA LOLASANA

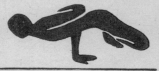

7

7. Start in the same manner as Lolasana, #6. Place right palm in front with fingers towards you on the ground — Forearm vertical — Bend forward and place abdomen on elbow — Balance body with the other arm at the back. Hold the position and then alternate to the other arm.

BENEFITS: — Elbow pressing into abdomen and liver increases the blood supply. Relieves chest and abdominal diseases. Reduces abdominal fat, piles and constipation. Helps evacuation of excretory system. Helps balance the body.

DHANURASANA
The Bow

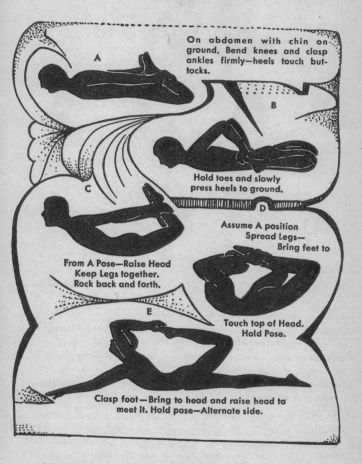

On abdomen with chin on ground. Bend knees and clasp ankles firmly—heels touch buttocks.

Hold toes and slowly press heels to ground.

From A Pose—Raise Head Keep Legs together. Rock back and forth.

Assume A position Spread Legs— Bring feet to

Touch top of Head. Hold Pose.

Clasp foot—Bring to head and raise head to meet it. Hold pose—Alternate side.

BENEFITS For All: — Greatly strengthens and develops entire spine, lumbar area, chest, legs, arms, head and neck. Stimulates circulation throughout body.

ANDHA MATSEDRASAN

Front   Back

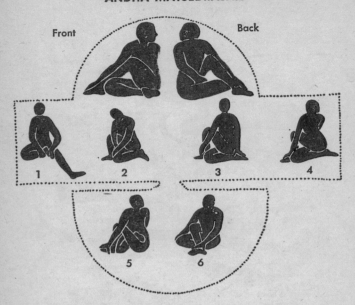

1. Assume the Half Lotus by bringing the right foot up with foot under left thigh.
2. Bring the left leg up and over the bent leg as far back as possible.
3. Bring right shoulder, right elbow and arm in front and around the left knee. With right hand, clasp the ankle of the left leg.
4. Twist body and head around and over the left shoulder as far as possible.

Hold this position. Breathe with regular rhythm — Concentrating — Meditating. Alternate to other side.

BENEFITS: — Twists the spine to two sides, twisting each vertebra, spinal column and sympathetic nervous system with gentle massaging action. Muscles of shoulders and abdomen are stretched and benefited. Constipation and dyspepsia are relieved. Liver, spleen and kidneys are stimulated. This Asana convulses and squeezes the aorta etc., giving the blood an extra push throughout the body.

5.-6. Foot is on top of thigh instead of flat against thigh. This is an advanced Asana and is mastered after practicing regular Half Twist.

ANJANEYASANA — Leg Split

BEGINNERS

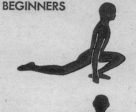

Inhale

A — Stretch leg back as far as you can, keeping foot on the floor.

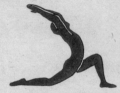

Retain Air

B — Turn body to the Front.

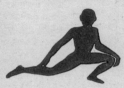

C — Raise arms above head. Slowly bend back — arching the back as far as possible.

Exhale

Relax

BENEFITS: — To stretch pelvic muscles and inner thighs, legs, spine, and torso.

ANJANEYASANA — Leg Split
ADVANCED VARIATIONS

Head to knee — Hands to toes.————

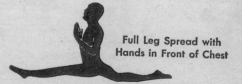

Full Leg Spread with Hands in Front of Chest

BENEFITS: — To stretch pelvic muscles and inner thighs, legs, spine, and torso.

KATIKASANA — Pelvic Pose

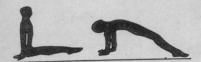

From sitting position with palms at the sides of hips.
Slowly straighten arms and raise pelvis.

SUPTA VAJRASAN— Stretching Spine

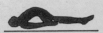

Hands under buttocks with palms on the ground. Raise body straight up. Roll head back. Chest is high. Hold.

KAMDHARASANA— Neck Bridge Pose

1. Arms crossed at chest. Knees bent. Heels at buttocks.
2. Raise hips. Roll slowly from shoulders to top of head.

URDHVA DHANURASANA — Raised Bow

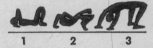

1. Draw feet to buttocks as you bend knees. Palms are opposite the shoulders.
2. Raise hips to make a bridge.
3. Straighten arms and legs. Hold position.

VARIATIONS

PRISTHASANA — Wheel Pose

CAKRASANA

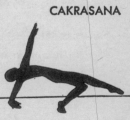

Alternate leg and arms.
Hold position a little longer with each attempt.

BENEFITS derived from exercises on this page: —
:Strengthens neck and torso. Stretches spine and hamstrings of legs.

TRIPADASANA — Three Footed Pose

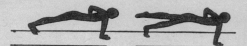

From Quadruped Pose — Raise one arm behind back. Eztend the leg of the same side straight out and up, parallel to the body to form a straight line. Hold this position. Repeat on other side.

BENEFITS: — Stretches and strengthens legs, arms and back.

Arm — Leg Pose — BAHU PADASANA

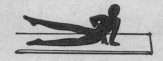

From Quadruped Pose — Turn on side, supporting body on foot and hand. Hold position. Repeat on other side.

Quadruped Pose — CATUSPADASANA

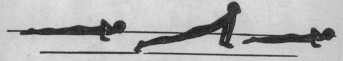

Inhale and   Hold Air.   Exhale and repeat.

Legs together. Hands parallel to shoulders. Straighten arms. Rise on toes.

BENEFITS: — Strengthens arms, legs stomach muscles and back.

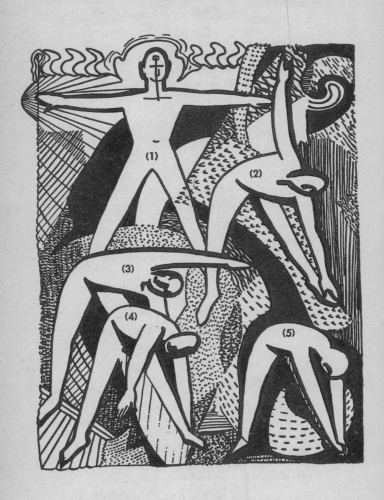

GRIVASANA — Neck Posture

BEGINNERS   **ADVANCED**

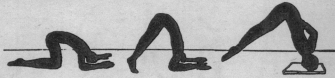

1
Kneel on ground
with feet together.
Arms close to head.

2
Straighten legs.
Roll to center of
Head. Hold position.

3
From pose #2 Bring
hands to back. Hold
pose.

BENEFITS: — Sends blood to head.

Pelvic Stretch
SUPTA VAJRASANA

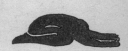

1   **2**   **3**

The pelvic stretch can be done as a
posture and held as in #2 or #3.

It is also an exercise if the three positions are taken without resting one after
the other.

Grivasana and Supta Vajrasana are
complementary positions to each other.

71

TRIKONASAN — Triangle Postures

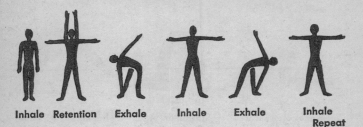

| Inhale | Retention | Exhale | Inhale | Exhale | Inhale Repeat |

Stand erect — Raise arms to the sides — then up — Turn body at waist — Bend down and touch opposite foot with hand. Repeat on the other side.

CHANDRASANA — Moon Postures

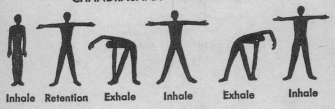

| Inhale | Retention | Exhale | Inhale | Exhale | Inhale |

Keep chest and face facing front — Bend at waist. Don't bend the knees.

TRIKONASAN

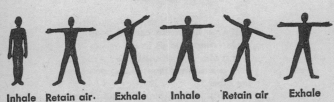

| Inhale | Retain air | Exhale | Inhale | Retain air | Exhale |

Repeat — Keep legs and arms straight. Head is turned with the body.

TRIKONASAN — Variations

TRIANGLE POSTURE
Facing Front

Exercises to reduce waist line.

CHANDRASANA —
Moon Posture
Looking Back

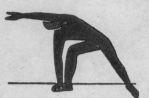

Right hand to right foot — Alternate.

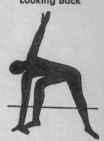

Right hand to left foot.

Waist Roll Twist

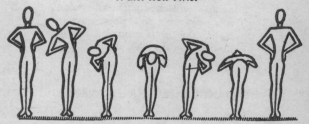

ARDHA CHANDRASANA — Moon Pose

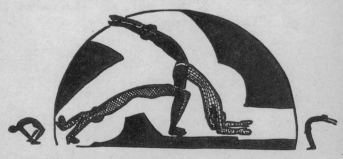

Bend back from Bent knees. Hold. Bend forward from Waist.

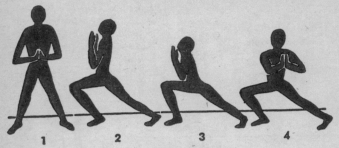

1   2   3   4

TECHNIQUE: — 1. Legs apart — Hands together — Palms touching. 2. Turn right — bend right knee. 3. Lean forward and down — keeping left leg straight. Hold pose. 4. Turn to front again — pushing right hand against left palm and left palm pushing against right palm in traction. Repeat the same on the other side.

PADANGUSHTASANA — Leg Raise

5. From 1, 2 then 3 (skipping #4) attain position #5 by raising leg and bending at waist — Hold — Rest and repeat on other side.

BENEFITS: — Stretches the muscles of the legs, spine, chest, back, neck, arms, wrists, ankles, feet and toes. Helps balance and poise.

UPRIGHT POSITION — TWIST

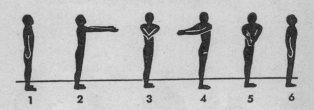

1. Inhale slowly.
2. Raise arms to shoulder level. Gaze at top of hands.
3.-4. Slowly twist arms to left as far as possible. Keep gaze on hands.
5.-6. Return to original position. Exhale. Repeat same on the right side.

BACK STRETCH

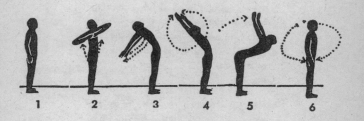

TECHNIQUE: — 1. Keep legs straight and hips to the front — Feet flat on the ground — or toes. 2.-3. Hands to chest — out and back — 4. Up over head and bend back as far as possible. 5. Bend forward — Arms are kept back. 6. Straighten up to #1.

PADA HASTHASAN — Head to Knee Pose

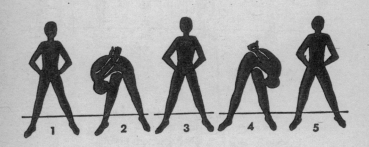

1. Legs three to four feet apart. Hold wrist behind back — Inhale.
2. Exhale as you bend slowly — turning body — Bring head to knee. Exhale.
3. Return to original position. Inhale.
4. Exhale as you bend slowly to the other side.
5. Repeat.

BENEFITS: — Stretch is felt in spine, waist, shoulders, legs, arms, neck, chest·and back. The blood is sent to all these parts and to the head. Helps keep the midriff streamlined.

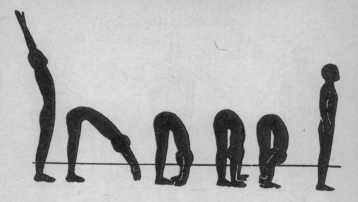

Knees stiff — Inhale as you stretch arms overhead.

Exhale as you reach forward and out — arms close to head.

Touch palms to the ground. Bring head to knees. Grasp ankles.

Return to original position.

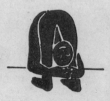

Bring head through legs — Clasp hands around ankles.

BENEFITS: — Stretch is felt in spine, waist, shoulders, legs, arms, neck, chest and back. The blood is sent to all these parts and to the head. Helps keep the midriff streamlined.

VATYANASANA

BEGINNERS ASANAS

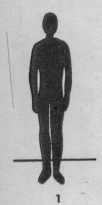

1

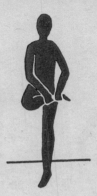

2

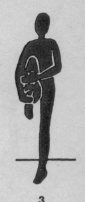

3

1. Relax — Focus eyes on a spot parallel to eye level.

2. Slowly bring foot up and hold ankle as long as comfortable.

3. Bring knee up. Press to body. Press ankle inward.

BELKA ASANA — Crane Pose

Advanced

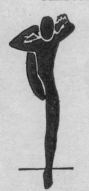

Elka Pada Pose

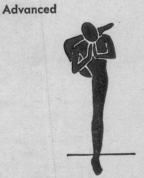

Elka Pada Sirasan

VATYANASANA

ELKA PADA HASTHASAN

UTTHA JANUSIRASANA

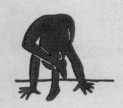

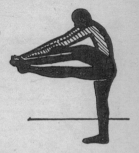

From Crane Pose Bend Down.

Bring leg straight front and up.
Hold foot with both hands.
Slowly bend at the waist. Exhale as head touches knee.

UTTHA PADAPRASARASAN

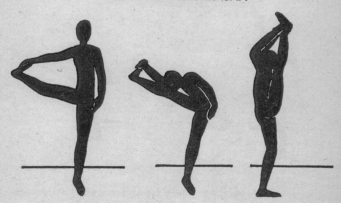

Out to Side.

Keep chest to the
front as you turn
head and put it on
the knee.

Leg overhead. Hold
with both hands.
Head to knee.

LORD MATARAJASON POSES

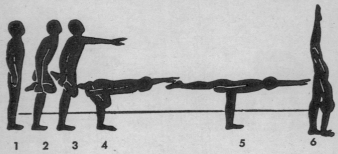

1   **2**   **3**   **4**   **5**   **6**

1. Stand erect.
2. Bend knee and hold ankle.
3. Press heel against buttocks.
4. Extend arm out straight. Bend slowly from waist.
5. Release ankle — extend leg and arm back. Hold pose.
6. Holding body in a straight line, bend down and rest palm on the ground in front of foot. Head to knee.

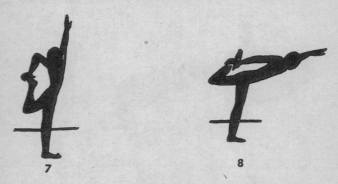

7   **8**

7. From position #3 — Bring leg and arm up. Hold pose.
8. From post #7 above — slowly bend forward.

Alternate sides on all these poses.

VRSHASAN —
Tree Posture

Leg Twisters

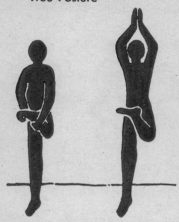

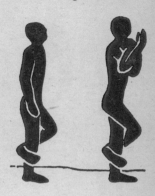

Bring foot up with both hands across the thigh of the other leg.

Raise arms over head and hold palms together. Hold pose as long as you are able.

Cross and encircle right leg in front and around left thigh and ankle.

One arm encircles the other arm. Palms are pressed together. Hold.

GARUDASANA

Eagle Pose

Alternate

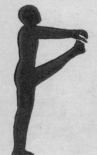

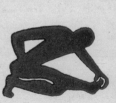

Focus eyes on a spot to assist control of balance. Hold foot. Keep leg straight.

Rise on toes and slowly lower body keeping the back and leg straight.

BENEFITS: — (Derived from these Asanas)

Makes the spine resilient. Tones up the nervous system. Helps natural peristaltic action in the colon. Strengthens balance control. Increases height.

URVASANA — Knee bending exercise

For Balance Control — Spine and Legs.

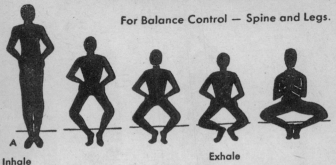

A

Inhale

Exhale

Rise on toes — Slowly bend knees — Focus on a spot.

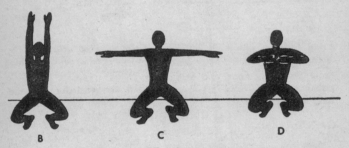

B   **C**   **D**

These are variations of hand positions.
Can be done as up — side and hands
on chest — in A fourth position.

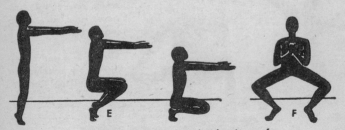

E   **F**

These are variations and side views of
above and have similar benefits. Breath
control is taken on up — released on
down.

PADANDGUSHTASANA — Tiptoe Pose

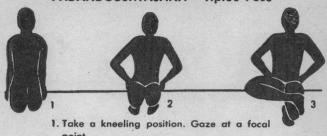

1. Take a kneeling position. Gaze at a focal point.
2. Raise knees slowly until you feel relaxed in this position. Balance on toes.
3. From #2 position — Raise leg and put foot over the thigh of other leg. Hold a few minutes then alternate to the other side.

ADVANCED: — Raise up and down in slow movements. Later — Springing up and down effect.

BENEFITS: — For tired muscles of ankles and toes. Beneficial for flat feet.

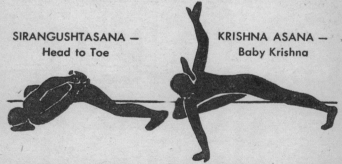

SIRANGUSHTASANA — Head to Toe

KRISHNA ASANA — Baby Krishna

Spread legs very far apart. Fold hands behind back and bend head to foot. Hold. Relax. Alternate sides.

One leg is passed over and behind head and wedged against the nape of neck. Balance is on one leg and opposite arm. Raise free arm. Alternate.

BENEFITS: — Stretches spine, neck, limbs and shoulders. All muscles are relaxed and benefited.

SUPTA — Forward Bend

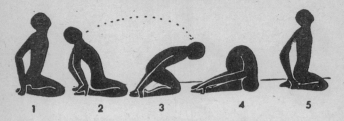

1. Kneel with palms of hands across soles of feet. Inhale.
2. Hold feet for support. Bend body and back as far back as possible.
3. Exhale — Lean slowly forward until head touches ground — close to knees.
4. Complete exhalation — Hold for a short time. Increase at each attempt.
5. Complete exhalation before inhaling and resuming original position.

LEG AND STOMACH EXERCISE

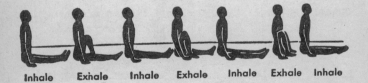

Inhale   Exhale   Inhale   Exhale   Inhale   Exhale   Inhale

Beginners leg exercise. Beneficial for stomach, waist, hips and legs.

BENEFITS for exercises on this page:—

Develops bust, chest, abdomen and upper back. Strengthens toes, feet, ankles and neck. Prevents lumbago and joint diseases. Removes tension and stiffness of body and limbs. Relieves gaseous disturbances, tightens hamstrings and stomach muscles.

FORWARD ROLL OR TUMBLESAULT

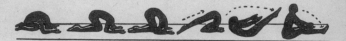

A fun exercise for the family with tremendous benefits.

TECHNIQUE: — Knees, arms and back are held very close together. Feet touching. Lift back and push hips over head.

STREAMLINE FOR THE LADIES

A

A — From back — Roll the hip then leg over — Top part of body follows— Keep rolling until you are again on the back. Repeat over and over again until tired.

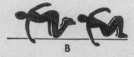

B

B — With knees bent — Swing hips only, to right, then left side. Head and shoulders remain flat.

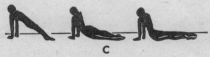

C

C — Rise up straight. Bounce left hip then right hip on the ground. Keep legs and knees straight throughout. The weight of the body is supported on straight arms and legs.

ARDHA KURMASAID — Hammock Swing

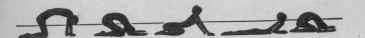

From kneeling position — Hunch back and lower to the heels. Stretch out and Hunch again.

Do the above exercises *with* or *without music*. Benefits are for internal organs, reducing the hips, waist, thighs and firming bust.

Recommended for women who wish to regain their youthful figure after child birth.

VARIATIONS

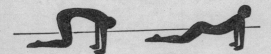

Exhale then Inhale. Arch your back — Like a cat.

Inhale on up. Exhale and lower the pelvis and abdomen.

DOLASANA — Swing Posture

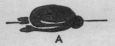

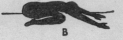

A — Head in front of knees. Arms close to sides.

B — Put head to chin straight out in front of head.

KAREN ANN'S ANIMALS — "Walk"

Fun Exercises for the Family

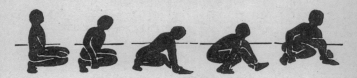

Holding ankles — Kneeling on toes —
Slowly bring one leg at a time out.
Weight is on the back leg and is trans-
ferred as you move forward. This is a
"Fun" exercise.

BENEFITS:— Benefits are the same as
above including muscle and back
strengthening.

Camel's Walk
Cat Stretch

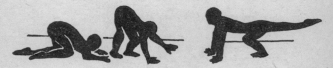

Frog
Dog Run

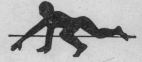

TECHNIQUE is the same as above except
that both knees are put on one and
the same arm. Hold pose a few seconds. Alternate to the other arm.

BENEFITS: — Benefits are the same as
above including muscle and back
strengthening.

BOW — DHANURASANA

ASANAS

Grasp Ankles   Lift and Rock
                Back and Forth

NAUKASANA — Boat Pose

Spread Legs Apart. Hold.
Exercise by rocking back and forth.

Swing High — Swing Low (To Music)

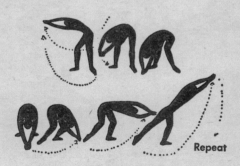

Repeat

— Alternate sides —

MANDUKASANA — Frog Pose

1. Sit on heels, in a knee bending position, on toes. Balance with the knees apart. Focus your eyes on a spot on the level with the head.

2. Put the palms of hands firmly on the ground, parallel to toes.

3. Rest knees on respective arms. Rise slowly from toes. Balance the body on the arms.

Besides the many benefits for various parts of the body this Asana is helpful for those having difficulty with the Head-stand.

PARSWA KAKASANA

VARIATION OF FROG POSE

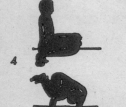

TECHNIQUE is the same as above except that both knees are put on one and the same arm. Hold pose a few seconds. Alternate to the other arm.

VAKRASANA — Curved Pose

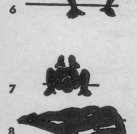

7. Hands are parallel to shoulders.

8. Put one hand between the thighs and cross ankles. Upper ankle is under the lower in an ankle lock. Slowly raise body in a straight line.

9. Balance weight and hold the position. Relax then alternate side.

BENEFITS: — The above Asanas relaxes and stretches entire body.

89

NERVE STIMULATION

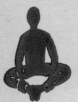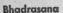

Bhadrasana **Bhadrasana** **Khanda Peeda** **Gorakaka Asana**
Ankle Knee Pose Ankle Twist Ankle Knee Pose

SAKTHI CHALINI

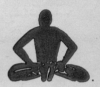

FOR FEET AND TOES

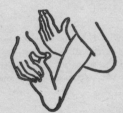

**Manipulate toes, heel and ankle
in all directions.**

Secretary's Leg and Foot Stretch

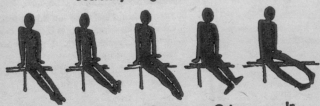

Down   **Up**   **Down**   **Out**   **In**

Very Slow — NECK EXERCISES — Closed Eyes

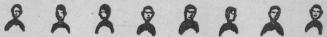

Inhale   Retain air   Exhale — Inhale   Retention of Breath — Exhale

Turn head slowly while you control breathing. Repeat.

HEAD TO SHOULDER

Inhale   Exhale   Inhale   Exhale   Inhale

Repeat

FORWARD — AND — BACK

   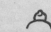

Inhale   Hold — Exhale   Inhale   Hold — Exhale   Inhale

Hold the down and the back positions.

Repeat

CIRCLE

Inhale   and   Hold   until   you get back to 1st position.

Repeat starting from alternate side.

HEAD PUSH — CLOSED EYES

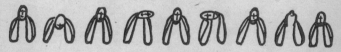

Inhale   Exhale   Inhale   Retain   Exhale   Retain   Inhale   Retain   Exhale

Clasp hands in back of neck at lower part of head. Elbows rest on table. Head is slowly, gently pressed down. Chin on chest. Hold then exhale. Return to front position. Head is pressed to shoulders, back and front.

BENEFITS: — Relieves stiffness and tensions around neck and upper spine.

ALTERNATING ARM SLAPS

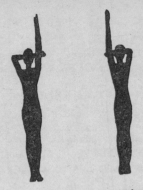

Raise one arm straight up. With the flat palm of the other hand slap the inner side of the up right arm with heavy, quick, stinging slaps.

ARM EXERCISES

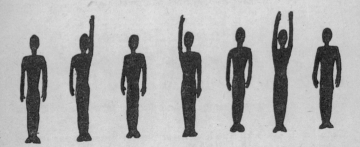

Inhale as you raise arm over head. Exhale as you lower the arm, or arms. Raise arm quickly, hold position then lower quickly. Repeat until tired.

BENEFITS: — For reducing fatty arms.

Push — Pull Traction for Breast and Upper Arms
for Women

Sit or Stand — Press Palms together.

Push to Right — use Traction with left.

Relax

Push to Left — use Traction with right.

Relax. Alternate Sides.

The same as above. With hands clasped.

The same as above. With arms over head.

Arms — Breast — Back
for Women

out
Inhale

up
Exhale

in
Inhale

out
Exhale

back
Repeat
Cycle

Hands are clasped behind neck and lower part of head.

BENEFITS: — Develops rounded curves by strengthening pectoral muscles. Also benefits the arms and back.

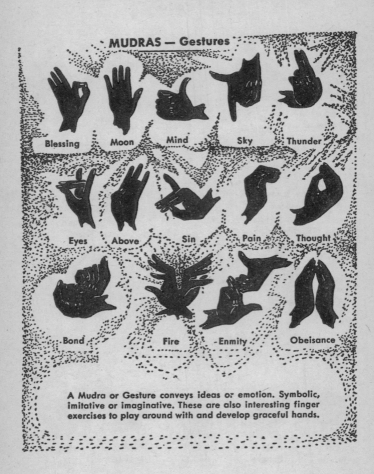

MUDRAS — Gestures

Blessing	Moon	Mind	Sky	Thunder
Eyes	Above	Sin	Pain	Thought
Bond		Fire	Enmity	Obeisance

A Mudra or Gesture conveys ideas or emotion. Symbolic, imitative or imaginative. These are also interesting finger exercises to play around with and develop graceful hands.

HAND — WRIST — FINGERS

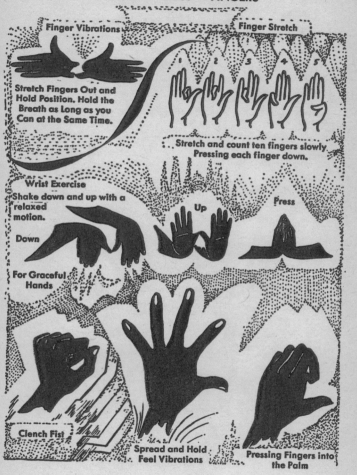

Finger Vibrations

Stretch Fingers Out and Hold Position. Hold the Breath as Long as you Can at the Same Time.

Finger Stretch

1 2 3 4 5

Stretch and count ten fingers slowly. Pressing each finger down.

Wrist Exercise

Shake down and up with a relaxed motion.

Down

Up

Press

For Graceful Hands

Clench Fist

Spread and Hold Feel Vibrations

Pressing Fingers into the Palm

SIMHASANA — Lion Pose

Imitate a Lion

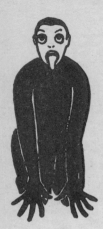

Kneel and sit back on heels.
Spread hands on knees.
Thrust tongue out as far as you can —
Mouth wide open.
Eyes opened very wide.
Look up — Breathe deeply.
Tense your body.

Touch tongue to Nose.

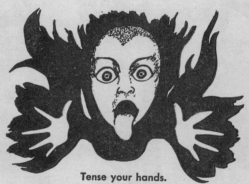

Tense your hands.
Thrust tongue out as far as you can —
Mouth wide open.
Eyes opened very wide.
Look up — Breathe deeply.

BENEFITS: — Tones up facial muscles, tongue, throat, tonsils and eyes. Stimulates circulation of blood throughout your body.

TRATAKUM — Training the Gaze

Eye Exercises

Circling the Eyes

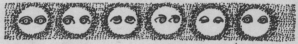

Front   Right   Up   Left   Down   Forward

Move eyes slowly around the room clockwise. Hold each position to one heart beat. Relax — Then reverse the exercise by starting towards the left.

BENEFITS: — Relieves tension and fatigue of eyes and eye strain. Strengthens optic nerves and muscles. Helps concentration of the mind.

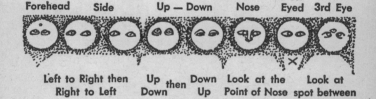

Forehead   Side   Up — Down   Nose   Cross-Eyed   3rd Eye

Left to Right then Right to Left   Up then Down   Down Up   Look at the Point of Nose   Look at spot between eye brows.

When fixation, suggestions and sensations (Samyamah — total concentration) are directed to the exterior surface of the body or to any external object, it is called Tratakum. Concentration with open eyes.

BENEFITS: — To control mental waves and check restlessness of the mind. Eye sight will improve. Good preparation for meditation.

97

TRATAKUM — Training the Gaze

SUGGESTIONS: — Select a quiet room in a comfortable Lotus posture or an easy chair. As you gaze, make suggestions such as "I control my mind and all mental waves." If eyes tire, rest them for a moment before repeating.

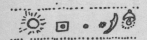
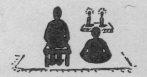

Gaze steadily at Disks, Spot, Star, Moon, Electric Light or Candles. Gaze at the Sun at Sunset or Sunrise.

For Concentration Power

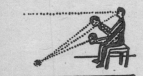

Gaze between two fingers. You will see the image of two more between. Or use candles. One or two.

Look and gaze — up and down — Far away.

The length of time you can do Tratakum will increase with practice.

NETI KRIYA — Nasal Cleansing

NETI is a Yoga process to clean the nasal passages. Destroys catarrh and other diseases of the nasal area. A soft cotton cord is used. Instruction should only be given by a qualified Yoga instructor.

Drinking water through the nose, the first thing on arising in the morning, has been found to be beneficial, and easier to learn to do. The water should be cold or lukewarm.

SWIMMING AND DIVING

Because swimming is not as natural an instinct to man as it is to fish and most quadrupeds, the ability to swim well is more of an art when it is scientifically taught. The method used by the American Red Cross in their aquatic schools has been perfected and developed from styles of swimming research, dating as far back as the year 1500. Competitive swimming and diving is mostly responsible for the speed and improved methods used to date. The Olympic meets and the vast interest shown, is proof of the desire of man for this sport. High divers leaving the diving board and flying through space have the beauty of birds, and underwater swimmers give competition to fish. Man is the most amazingly versatile creature both in the air and in the water.

Age is no limitation. No tension or strain is used. By eliminating the fear of water, one strengthens his personality and improves his health.

Combining as many of the Hatha Yoga exercises as lends itself to the buoyancy of the water, Dr. Mishra and his students, added swimming instructions and Water Hatha Yoga to their yearly Yoga Convocations.

The benefits for rejuvenation of mind and body are unlimited. One should concentrate on studying each movement as illustrated.

Whenever possible, the breathing exercises as used in Hatha Yoga, are used in the Water Hatha Yoga. The body can be more relaxed in the water by its own buoyancy. The mirrored effect of the water, the rays of the sun's penetration, and Asanas along with meditation and Tratakum, is of great advantage.

CAUTION

At no time, as beginner or advanced swimmer, extend the length of time of holding the breath under water to the danger point.

ACKNOWLEDGMENT

Instructions regarding the correct methods as illustrated in the following pages were edited by my former instructor:

Mr. Leroy C. Peters, Executive Director of the Westchester County Chapter-American Red Cross, White Plains, New York.

For further swimming material consult the American Red Cross, Safety Services and Water Safety for such material as "Swimming and Diving," "Life Saving and Water Safety," and instructor's manuals.

MENTAL PICTURES: FOR FLOATING

Floating Experiments for Non-swimmers

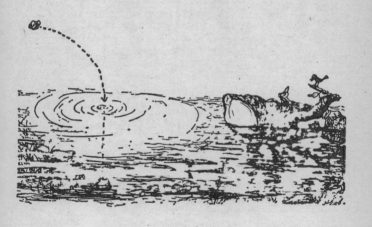

MENTAL PICTURES: — Drop a pebble or rock into the water — Watch it sink. Throw a log or stick out and watch it float on the water. The tremendous log floats because it holds *air*. The more relaxed we are the more air we hold.

Don't turn to stone by fear . . . Be buoyant by *relaxing*.

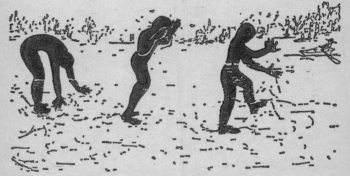

PHYSICAL ADJUSTMENT

a. Enter water gradually — to the knees — wet wrists.

b. To the hips — wet face, back of neck and chest.

c. Submerge entire body — kicking, splashing and jumping up and down happily.

MENTAL PREPARATION

Shock of cold water will cause tenseness.

A relaxed approach in learning eliminates fear and helps co-ordination.

Fear causes irregular breathing which will tire us unnecessarily.

The more enjoyable the learning, the faster we master new skills.

SAFETY AND GOOD SENSE

Always have a buddy with you.

Adjust to water by gradually submerging body.

Cooling the body temperature to avoid shock.

FLOATING EXERCISES
For Lake and Beach

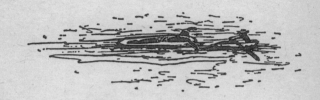

Throw Row Go

Safety Devices
Towel
Life Buoy
Bamboo Pole

Buoyancy and Breathing

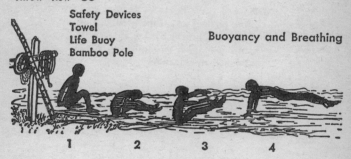

1.   2.   3.   4.

1. Sit on the bottom, then gradually move forward until your hips are covered with water. Feel the buoyancy of the water by raising legs and putting palms on top or just beneath the water.
2. Inhale — Put face down into water and blow bubbles as you exhale through the mouth. Repeat putting face into water after inhaling and count to see how long you can do this, increasing the time gradually.
3. Move forward slowly until the water covers body up to chest. Allow legs to float.
4. Rest the weight of body on stiff arms and allow legs and hips to float up relaxed and naturally.

HORIZONTAL BACK FLOAT
On a Beach or Shallow Part of Pool

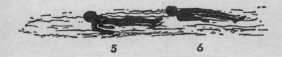

5   **6**

5. From relaxed position (as in #4 above) with face out of water, allow hips to float higher than the legs.

6. Release arms from the bottom and bring or float up off the ground. This exercise will occur by the body's natural buoyancy if the body and mind is completely relaxed.

SAFETY DEVICES
At the Pool-Floating

Bamboo Pole   Life Buoy

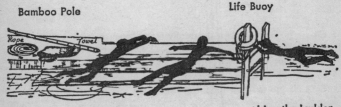

Using the Steps   Using the Ladder

Rest arms on a step just above the waterline. Allow the legs to float up. Observe the body's buoyancy. Try both positions — on back and face down. Exhale out into the water.

BUOYANCY

FLOATING ON BACK

Finding the body's natural buoyancy.

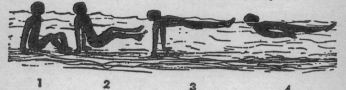

1 2 3 4

1. Sit on the bottom with the water up to chin.
2. Place hands to rear of hips.
3. Relax and allow legs and hips to float up by themselves. Bring head back and stiffen arms. Chest is raised up.
4. When completely relaxed, slowly remove arms to the sides. Hold this floating pose until you feel as relaxed as in bed.

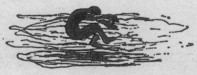

5

5. In recovery, to regain footing, bend at the waist as you push down with the palms of hands. Bring the head down at the same time.

This is the basis for all back strokes. Achieve this and the rest is systematic.

PRONE FLOATING

Finding the body's natural buoyancy.

Relate
with Hatha Yoga
PASCHIMOTTANASAN —
(Cobra Pose)

PRANAYAMA —
(Breath Control)

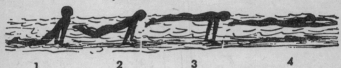

1   2   3   4

1. Kneel in the water to the depth of neck or shoulders.
2. Inhale and put face down into the water as you let legs and hips float up.
3. Round the back slightly.
4. Gently release hands from the bottom and bring hands together in front of head. Stretch out on the water, but do not stiffen. Relax completely as if in bed.

To regain footing

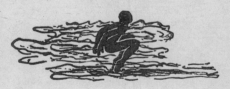

Exhale in #4 as you lift head and bend knees to chest and at the waist. Bring feet down.

BEGINNERS SKILLS

Prone Float from Standing Position.

A — Water Depth — to Hips   Associate with Breath Control
                                          Yoga — Pranayama

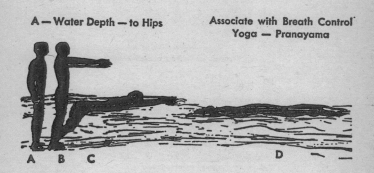

A   B   C   D

B — Inhale. With knees slightly bent, stretch forward face down and hands together.

D — Exhale slowly or hold breath in this position. Breath control is your choice.

CONCENTRATE: — Relaxing and increasing the length of time.

Prone Glide from the Side of Pool.

Associate with Yoga Pranayama.

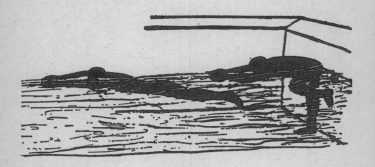

One foot flat against the side of the pool. The other foot is flat on the floor. Bend from the waist, arms out and thumbs locked. Inhale. Hold breath as you push away from wall. Glide relaxed until you need fresh air. Repeat all except exhale slowly into water before you regain footing.

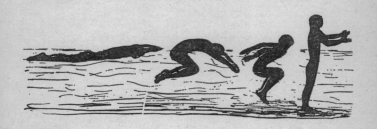

From floating position — bend at the waist — press palms against the water. Raise head up and back. Straighten legs and bring arms up. If this is done slowly and relaxed with concentration, you will have no trouble.

All non-swimmers skills and exercises should be mastered with ease and complete relaxation before learning styles of swimming strokes. This will assure safety and tireless swimming.

NON-SWIMMERS SKILLS

Flutter Kick

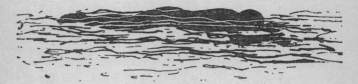

Lie in water just covering body. Weight is on arms in front of head.

Shallow Water

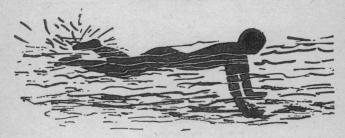

Straighten arms in shallow water. With relaxed legs, float then kick from the hips, with small *slaps* *down* at the water with the instep of foot.

First try this with head out of. water. Then inhale and put face down into the water.

CONCENTRATE ON:

I am relaxed.
From the hips — relaxed knees.
Slap down with the instep of foot.

This will result in tireless swimming and speed later on.

NON-SWIMMERS SKILLS

At the Pool

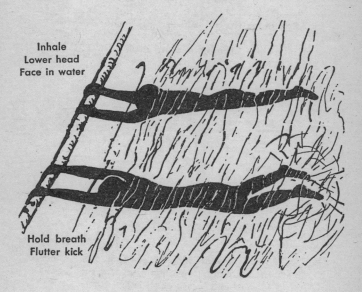

Inhale
Lower head
Face in water

Hold breath
Flutter kick

Breath Control Exercises

Hold rail at the pool with arms parallel to shoulders.

Inhale and hold breath under the water. Increase length of time with practice.

Repeat the above and add the Flutter Kick.

CONCENTRATE ON:
   I am relaxed.
   From the hips — relaxed knees.
   Slap down with the instep of foot.
This will result in tireless swimming and speed later on.

NON-SWIMMERS SKILLS

Breathing Co-ordination with Front Overarm.

(One complete stroke)

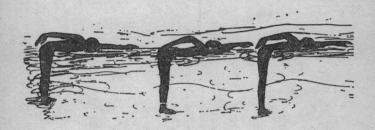

Stand in waist high water. One arm
straight back, the other arm straight
forward and face is down in the water.
As you bring the outstretched arm
straight down and the back arm up and
over, with a bent elbow, let the head
follow up. Take a breath of air through
the mouth. As the raised arm is lowered, the head returns down with the
roll of the shoulders, by itself. Exhale
the air and repeat cycle. See American
Crawl.

BEGINNERS SKILLS

Back Float

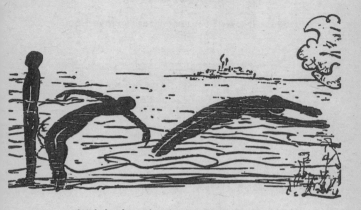

With back to the shore, in water waist or shoulder high. Spread arms out and slowly bend back until you have your shoulders, arms and head in the water. Allow legs to float off the ground. Stretch arms over head and straighten legs.

Breathe through the mouth. One must be completely relaxed to float correctly. Concentrate on the water as a soft bed that will hold you up.

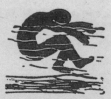

To recover footing
Bend head to chest. Bend at the waist. Touch hand to toes.

BEGINNERS SKILLS

The Roll Over from Back Float to Prone Float.

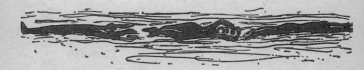

From the Back Float — Turn head face down into the water. Bring arm and leg up, back and around at the same time. Do this slowly with relaxed movements.

The Roll Over from Front Float to the Back Float.

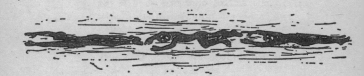

From the Front Float (or Face Down Float) bring arm and leg of the same side, back and around to the other side. Lead the turn with the head first. Do this slowly.

BEGINNERS SKILLS
Jelly Fish Float

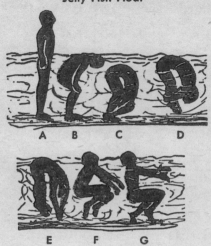

A   B   C   D

E   F   G

A — Stand in water up to the waist. Inhale a small amount of air.

B — With hands on knees put your face in the water.

C — Slowly lower hands and head until you grasp ankles.

D — Float up holding ankles. If you are completely relaxed this will be the natural reaction to the buoyancy of your body.

To regain standing position from prone float

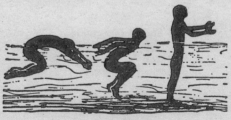

E — Release ankles and raise head. (From D above)

F — Straighten legs and feet will touch the bottom. Hands may assist by palms pushing down on the water.

BEGINNERS SKILLS

YOGA WATER PRANAYAMA — PADA HASTHASAN

Jelly Fish Float

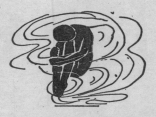

Hold knees against chest. Head to knees. You may retain this position as long as you can.

VARIATION: — Roll from side to side.

WATER HATHA YOGA

Spine and Leg Stretch

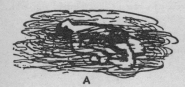 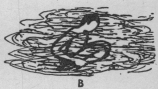

A   B

A — From back floating position — Very slowly grasp ankles behind the back. Slowly press heels back against your back, without straining.

B — Bend forward slowly, heels touching buttocks.

While learning, extreme caution is necessary as the spine is involved.

Benefits can be upset by tension or speed.

BEGINNERS SKILLS

PRONE GLIDE AND FLUTTER KICK

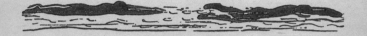

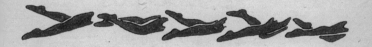

Kick is from the hips with relaxed legs. Slap down on the surface of the water with the instep of the foot. Short, quick strokes are faster and not as tiring as big ones.

Start with the prone glide, relax then flutter kick.

BEGINNERS SKILLS

FINNING AND SCULLING

Short arm strokes on back.

Series of little pushing or half sculling
movements of the hands.

Resting stroke of churning movements of
legs moving gently up and down.

KICK GLIDE ON BACK

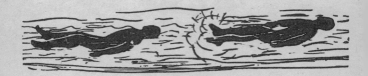

From a very relaxed back float. Inhaling
and exhaling through mouth.

Legs are pedalled with soles of feet
pushing down and backward on the
down stroke.

The instep of foot is spooning the water
up and backward on the upstroke.

FLOATING EXERCISES

Treading Water in an Upright Position

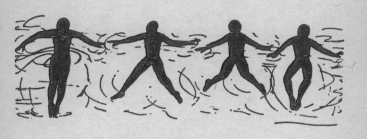

With head and neck above the water —
Breathe through the mouth.
A slightly forward and bent position of
the trunk is assumed.

Arms may be held in front of body or
to the side, just beneath the surface of
the water. Legs are beneath the body in
a crouching position from which the
stroke is delivered. A motion similar to
an egg beater can be used with hands
and feet or a short running motion of the
feet and pushing down with the palms
of the hands on the surface of the water.

SCISSORS KICK

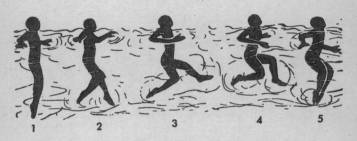

A slightly forward and bent posture is assumed.

With head and neck above the water — Breathe through the mouth.

Legs are spread, one in front and one in back, similar to a scissors.

Slowly bring legs as far back and forward as possible.

Snap legs together in a very fast stroke and hold together for a short rest with legs and body straight.

The kick is outward and down.

1. Completion of the rotation of the legs.
2. Is the ending and beginning of the stroke.

ELEMENTARY BACK STROKE

Start from horizontal Back Float with the arms
at the sides and chin tucked in and down.

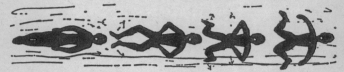

Begin Inhaling   Complete Inhalation

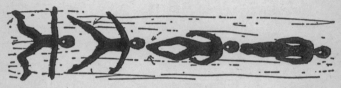

Hold Air — Begin Exhalation — Complete Exhalation.   Repeat Cycle.
Rest Position.

BREATHING: — Breathe through the mouth. Inhale as arms are being
raised to shoulder position. Exhale with the down thrust of the arms
to the sides.

ARMS: — The hands are rotated when they reach the shoulders with
the fingers facing outward. Catch the water and, like oars, pull
forcefully down with a broad sweeping stroke.

LEGS: — From legs together, slowly bring knees out to the sides with
the soles of the feet facing each other. Spread legs out as far as
possible with knees straight, then snap together with as much power
as you can. Hold together in the long glide.

RHYTHM: — Spread the legs and arms as slowly as possible, so as not
to stop the momentum, snapping the legs together and then holding
this position in a long glide should have a mental rhythm as, "Open,
open, open, snap together hold, hold and hold. With a long glide."
A count of three, one and then as many counts as the power of the
stroke gives you.

HEAD: — The chin is on the chest or a little above according to the
buoyancy of the body.

BREAST STROKE

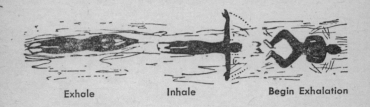

Exhale   Inhale   Begin Exhalation

Horizontal position — Relaxed Glide Float.

Arms are pulled to sides, horizontal to shoulder level. Legs are spread slowly to assume the recovery position. Hands are brought together at chest from shoulder level.

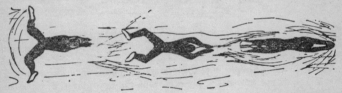

Recovery Position   Long Glide Rest Position

Continue Exhalation until momentum of long Glide begins to lose forward movement.

BREATHING is rhythmic and co-ordinated with the stroke. When the completion of the long glide is approached, the face is lifted and inhalation started and continued through the leg thrust and glide.

LEGS and ARMS: — Arms are pulled horizontally to the level of the shoulders then brought together at the chest for the recovery position and feet begin to draw together and out at about hip level.

BREAST STROKE

LEGS are lashed out and around to starting position where the long
   glide is made.

ARMS are fully extended in front of the head and legs together in
   the Glide.

BREAST STROKE KICK

Top View

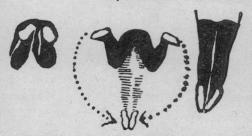

Draw legs up together with the soles facing each
other. Spread legs out slowly as far as you can in
the Recovery position. With toes pointing out,
thrust legs together with a fast powerful stroke.

Side View

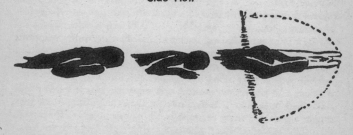

Starting at the chest and keeping palms together extend hands and
arms in front of head. Movement is like front dive. Hands are brought
to shoulder level with a fast, powerful pull and then slowly brought
to chest.

AMERICAN CRAWL

When learning, start from a relaxed face down float. The breathing is through the mouth. The head is in line with the spine. Body position is based on individual physical structure and buoyancy.

HAND-OVER-HAND STROKE

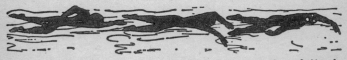

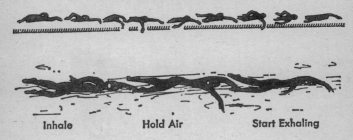

| Inhale | Hold Air | Start Exhaling |

| Continue Exhaling | Complete Exhalation | Inhale through Mouth |

ARMS: — Arm stroke is divided into two parts; the pull and the recovery. Entry is followed by extension and the catch is delayed. The recovery is more rapid. Extend the hand and allow it to drift downward several inches below the surface as the body rides over it by its own momentum. Drop hand, catch with a slightly cupped hand and pull through with a bent elbow drawing to the side of the hip. As the drawing arm passes the vertical arm near the hip, it relaxes and drifts back to the hip. It is then quickly drawn out of the water with a high elbow and flung forward as rapidly as possible. The arm is then fully extended, hand enters the water just beyond the head while the elbow is still high. Rest extended arm beneath the surface of the water for an appreciable interval before the next stroke begins.

AMERICAN CRAWL

LEGS: — The legs are close together and are extended just below the surface of the water. The knees are relaxed throughout the Flutter Kick with a vigorous beat of the shin and instep on the surface of the water. The kick is from the hip. This keeps the body horizontal and provides auxiliary propulsion.

HEAD: — The head is turned to one side only and face down. Find your natural side by experimenting. When the right arm is extended in a forward gliding position, the face is rotated (not lifted) to the left until nose and mouth are just above the surface. Inhale, then when the left arm is in recovering position it will turn the face down and forward for exhalation.

BREATHING: — Breathing should be a regular exchange of air and should not disrupt the rhythmic stroking or loss of balance. Air is gulped through the mouth and exhaled into the water as the head is automatically turned down.

BODY: — The back has a slightly rounded effect because of the submersion of the head, draw of the arms and hip position. During the arm glide the body is more streamlined.

CO-ORDINATION: — Perfect each part of the American Crawl as above, then try for co-ordination. Start with the glide float, kick, arms and then add the breathing with the head turn. Combined action of arms and legs come by practice.

SIDE STROKE

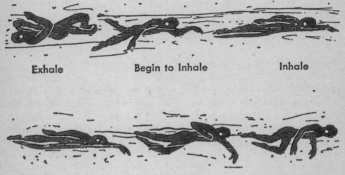

Exhale   Begin to Inhale   Inhale

Begin to Exhale   Exhale   Repeat Cycle

POSITION: — The body remains constantly in a side horizontal position near the surface with the back flat. The side of the head is submerged and in line with the spine. The legs are slightly lower than the head.

ARMS: — In starting position on the side, the lower arm is extended straight beyond the head, the cheek is rested on the extended shoulder. The upper arm is extended along the side with the palm resting on the thigh.

LEGS: — In starting the legs are extended backward, close together and with the toes pointed.

ARMS-LEGS: — To begin the stroke the lower arm catches the water and starts to pull straight down and the upper arm and legs begin to recover. As the lower arm completes its pull and starts to bend upward to recover, the upper arm and legs catch simultaneously, and drive through to complete the stroking movement; the lower arm meantime returning to its original extended position for the long glide which follows upon the completion of the stroke.

BREATHING: — The breath is taken through the mouth during the pull of the lower arm and exhaled as the upper arm delivers its thrust and throughout the glide. The breathing is done through the half open mouth in rhythm with the stroking.

POWER: — The power of the stroke is in the combined thrust of the legs and arm pull of the lower arm from the shoulder to just before it reaches the side of the hip.

RHYTHM: — Concentrate on; open legs very slowly, spread, prepare and snap legs together with speed and force. Co-ordinate the arms and breathing to this as described above. The rest glide position should be held until the momentum forward begins to slacken, then slowly start the next cycle.

OVERARM SIDE STROKE

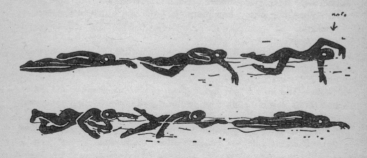

This stroke, in all respect, is the same as the Side Stroke except for the over arm reach past the head.

BACK CRAWL

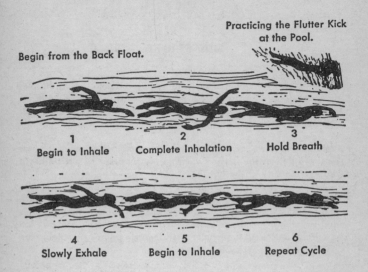

Practicing the Flutter Kick at the Pool.

Begin from the Back Float.

1 Begin to Inhale   **2** Complete Inhalation   **3** Hold Breath

4 Slowly Exhale   **5** Begin to Inhale   **6** Repeat Cycle

LEGS:—
1. Use the Flutter Kick. Ankles are kept relaxed. The big toes touch lightly as they pass when learning. Later the big toes just miss in passing.

CHIN: — Keep head and chin down and forward. Chin may also be kept on chest.

HANDS: — The little finger leads down as the hand enters the water and the thumb is up, pointing to the sky. Hands are slightly cupped in the pull down.
2.-3. Press the hand down parallel to the body as you pull arm straight down from the extended position above the head.

ARM: — One arm is always extended as the other arm is pulling down.
4.-5.-6. In the recovery, turn arm as the hand reaches the side of the body so that the palm faces away from the body. Toss the arm back with a relaxed motion up over the head.

BENEFITS: — The entire body is used in this technique of swimming. Stretching, relaxing and streamlining with the added benefits of water and Sun.

TRUDGEN STROKE

A racing stroke in which a double overarm motion is used and the legs execute a scissors kick.

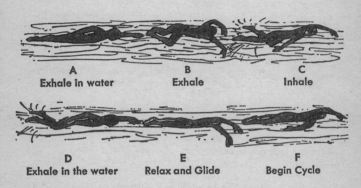

A	B	C
Exhale in water	Exhale	Inhale

D	E	F
Exhale in the water	Relax and Glide	Begin Cycle

LEGS: — A single Scissors stroke of the legs. As illustrated below.

ARMS: — The arm on one side strokes along while the other arm pull is combined with scissors kick of the legs.

BREATH: — The breath is taken at the height of the stroke which is during arm pull as the head is out of the water.

SCISSORS KICK

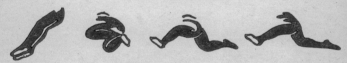

Open legs very slowly like a scissors. Legs are relaxed while opening them out as far as possible then snapped together with great force. Hold legs together and glide until momentum begins to lose power then repeat cycle.

TRUDGEN CRAWL STROKE

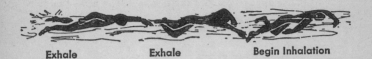

Exhale   Exhale   Begin Inhalation

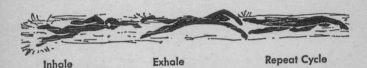

Inhale   Exhale   Repeat Cycle

LEGS: — Flutter kicks after each scissors kick. The flutter kick is used where the legs are held together for a glide in the above Trudgen Stroke.

ARMS: — The arm stroke and breathing is the same as American Crawl and Trudgen Stroke.

FLUTTER KICK

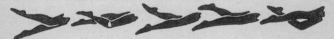

The kick is from a relaxed leg, loose ankle and starts from the hip with a slight bend at the knee.

SCISSORS KICK

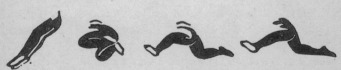

Open legs very slowly like a scissors. Legs are relaxed while opening them out as far as possible then snapped together with great force. Hold legs together and glide until momentum begins to lose power then repeat cycle.

BUTTERFLY

Free Style Swimming

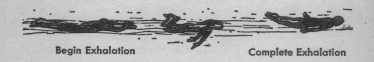

Begin Exhalation   Complete Exhalation

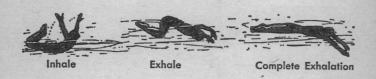

Inhale   Exhale   Complete Exhalation

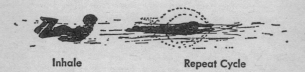

Inhale   Repeat Cycle

LEGS: — Dolphin kick. Feet together. The thrust is down from the knees.

ARMS: — Arms are kept close to the body and worked together in a complete circle.

BREATHING: — Air is gulped through the mouth in co-ordination with the rise and push down of the body.

BENEFITS: — Are similar to Hatha Yoga Salabhasan and Locust Pose.

INVERTED BREAST STROKE

Start from the Back Float.

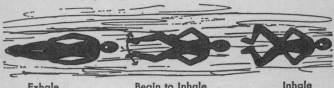

Exhale   Begin to Inhale   Inhale

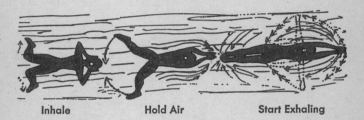

Inhale   Hold Air   Start Exhaling

ARMS: — From the Back Float with arms at the sides. Slowly bring arms up over head by drawing hands, with palms facing in, along the body.

*LEGS:— The legs are opened out at the same time with the soles of the feet facing each other. Knees come out to the sides then spread out as far as possible very slowly, to prepare for a fast snap together.

GLIDE: — Hold the complete stretched position until the height of its momentum, then snap hands to the sides with as much force and power as you can. Repeat cycle.

BREAST STROKE KICK

Practice the Frog Kick at the Pool

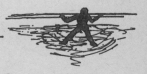

*(LEGS): — Open wide very slowly —
Hold — and Snap Together

BEGINNERS DIVING
FIVE PROGRESSIVE STEPS

1. Sit and Roll Over.   **2. On one knee — Roll Over.**   **3. Stand — Roll Over.**

CAUTION: — Hands should be extended and out in front of head at all times.

Lock thumbs and keep arms close to ears. Inhale through the mouth just before you roll over the edge.

5. **Beginners Dive** — Stand with toes over edge of the pool. Raise arms over head and bend knees. Spring up, out and down.

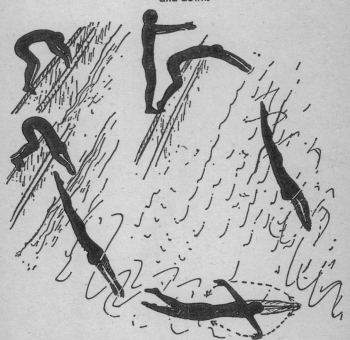

4. **Standing Push Off.** Keep head down, arms close to head with thumbs locked. Roll toes over the edge of the pool. Push off with the toes and straighten the knees.

Keep head down until you are ready to regain the surface.

BEGINNERS DIVING APPROACH
From the Board

Running FRONT HEADER from the SPRINGBOARD

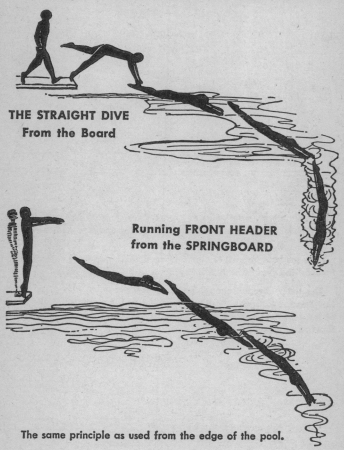

THE STRAIGHT DIVE
From the Board

Running FRONT HEADER
from the SPRINGBOARD

The same principle as used from the edge of the pool.

THE APPROACH

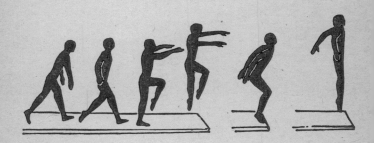

Stand erect with arms relaxed at the sides. From "inboard" end of board start the run along the board in evenly spaced, medium length strides.

One stride from back of the "outboard" end leap from one foot and land on the toes of both feet just back of the leading edge.

The jump (Hurdle) should be high and vigorous with arms timed to swing forward with the leap. Your weight, as you land on the balls of the feet, bends the board downward. In the rebound swing arms forward and upward.

SURFACE DIVE — FEET FOREMOST

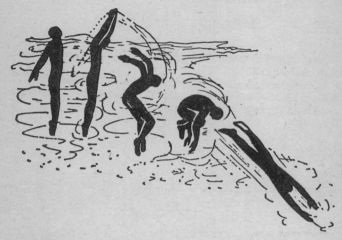

The same principle is used as in the Jacknife Surface Dive
except that the breath is taken with the head upright.

WITH SHORT FLUTTER KICKS

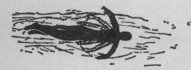

WITH SCISSORS KICK

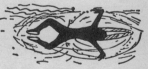

UNDERWATER SWIMMING

JACKKNIFE SURFACE DIVE

From the Crawl or Breast Stroke. Exhale through the nose and inhale through the mouth.

Use the Jackknife Surface Dive or Feet foremost Surface Dive. To surface, lift the head and reach upward. While swimming underwater use Breast Stroke kick or flutter kick.

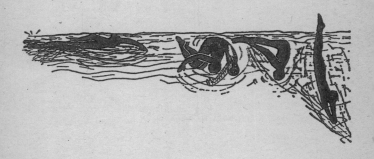

Using any swim stroke along the surface of the water, face downward, having some forward momentum, take a breath from the side and with a spreading movement of the arms the body is angled downward, the legs still on the surface of the water.

The legs are then lifted above the surface sharply until the body and legs are in one line.

The arms circle outward and downward. Use a Breast Stroke arm and either a short flutter kick or Breast Stroke kick.

To regain the surface, lift the head and press down with the palms against the water.

WATER — HATHA YOGA — EXERCISES

WRIST EXERCISES

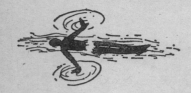

Use hands as
little oars.

Paddle back then paddle
forward.

TWISTING THE HIPS

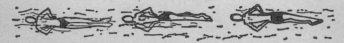

Float. Keep shoulders and chest up. Turn hips right and left.

ARM EXERCISES

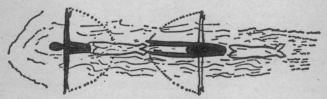

Inhale as arms are raised.

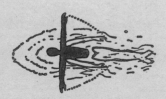

Exhale on Down.

CARTWHEEL

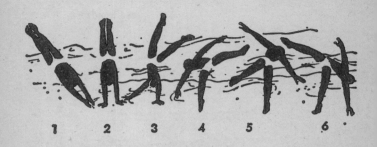

1   2   3   4   5   6

Dive to bottom with hands extended.
Water should not be over your head.

ROLLING

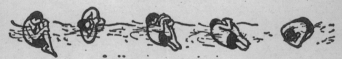

Clasp knees to chest. Chin to knees. Just roll.

SPINAL STRETCH

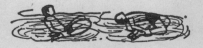

CAUTION: — Must be done extremely slowly for the first few times.
Grasp ankles with hands and draw heels to buttocks very slowly. At
the same time chest up and head back. Concentrate on feeling every
vertebra being stretched. Hold position, breathing deeply.

WATER — HATHA YOGA
FOR LAND OR DIVING BOARD

FROM BOARD

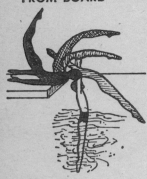

Stiffen body and throw legs overhead. Keep hands raised overhead until you want to rise. By lowering arms and pushing down with the palms you stop your feet first dive.

SALABHASAN — LOCUST
on Mat

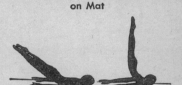

Inhale and slowly raise both legs.

VRISCHIKASAN — SCORPION

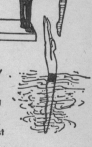

HAND STAND ASANA

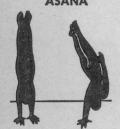

FROM BOARD

Drop legs slowly overhead—holding body and arms in a straight line. Hold this until you wish to rise. By lowering arms under water, you stop your feet first dive. Press hands down against the water at the same time.

More advanced swimmers and divers are able to enter the water this way in a regular Front Somersault dive. One must first learn the dive before the Hand Stand is added to it.

THE SWAN DIVE.

THE BACK DIVE

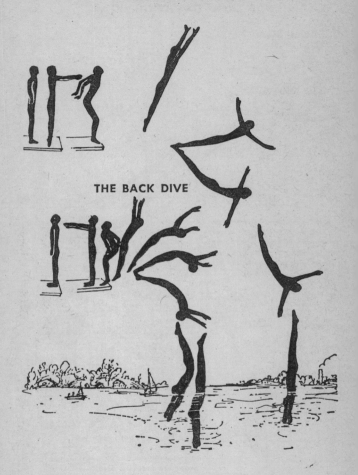

INTERPRETIVE — RHYTHMIC
DANCING

Where one is free to Let Go
and Express the Love of Music
and creative interpretations
of what they Feel, is Yoga.

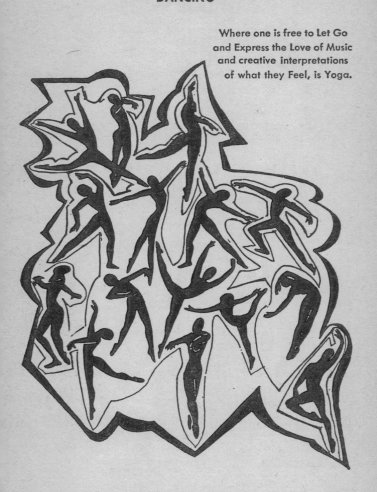

BEGINNERS

Pelvic Push and Raise removes Stiffness of Hips — Legs

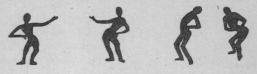

Twist movements definitely loosen the
muscles and releases suppressed energy.

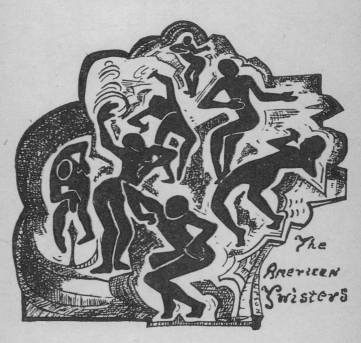